CW01390865

UNISLIM

The 30-Day Diet

UNiSLiM

The 30-Day Diet

over 75 easy & delicious recipes

Lose Weight & Improve Your Gut Health

Fiona Gratzer

EBURY PRESS

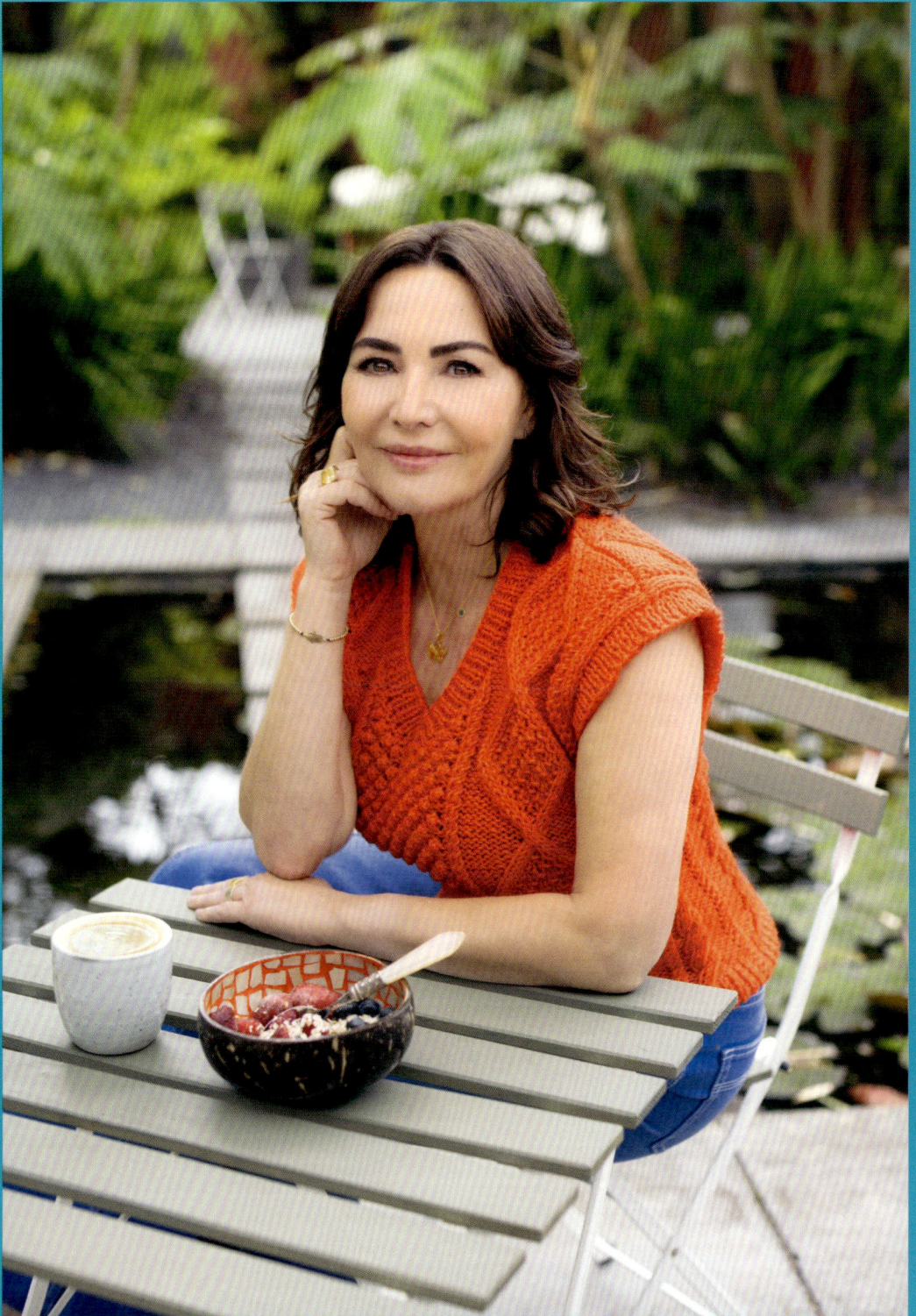

FOREWORD

It's no exaggeration to say that food has always played a major role in my life. My dad was once arrested for smuggling yogurt across the border in Northern Ireland, and my mum made her own kefir and pickled her own beetroot back in the 1970s, long before anyone was talking about gut health. My passionate, entrepreneurial parents pioneered Ireland's first weight-loss club, Unislim, in 1972, and I am honoured to be continuing their legacy.

When I was studying in Dublin, I'd spend my summers working for Unislim, but as soon as I got my degree I bolted to the airport to travel the world, footloose and fancy-free. As fate would have it, I fell in love within two weeks of starting my big adventure, having met my future husband, Uwe, on a secluded beach on a small island in Malaysia. This changed everything.

Uwe, who was from Austria, moved to Dublin and we soon got married. My work at Unislim went from being a summer job to becoming my full-time passion. I loved it so much that I studied nutrition and kept up to date with all the recent findings in the field. Meanwhile, Uwe had introduced me to the traditional food of Austria, including pickled, fermented and preserved foods – all good-gut favourites that continue to influence my eating today.

I was fit, active and healthy. I had two gorgeous children, I had run a marathon, and I'd ticked a few boxes off my bucket list. Life was fantastic.

However, tragedy struck in 2015, when I lost Uwe in a motorbike accident after 23 years together. In the wake of this immense loss, I experienced unexplained pains. After numerous MRI scans and consultations, these were eventually attributed to stress-induced referred pain. This personal experience showed me how deeply our emotions can affect our physical health – often, we may appear fine on the outside while fighting a battle within.

I was living with constant pain, but couldn't find any way to solve it. As chance would have it, I attended a wellness conference in America, and this inspired me to join the dots. I needed to rebalance my life and find ways to reduce stress. So, I took up yoga, started meditation and, in an effort to reduce inflammation in my body, I started eating more gut-friendly foods.

Ultimately, this inspired me to continue studying in this area, and I became a personal trainer and fitness instructor.

These days my health is back, I'm more energised, and I feel empowered knowing I can choose good foods for my gut health and wellbeing. My personal journey has led me to this book, the *30-Day Diet*, where small (micro) changes to your lifestyle can yield big gains for your gut health and happiness.

Helping people is my passion, and each year we transform thousands of members' lives through Unislim. Knowing that I've helped even one person live a healthier life gives me goosebumps. With this book, I've combined over three decades' worth of my experience, knowledge and study to create a gut-healthy guide to enhance your wellbeing, and my hope is that it will inspire you to embrace a life of greater health and happiness.

Fiona x

INTRODUCING THE 30-DAY DIET

WELCOME

You've just taken your first step towards becoming a happier, healthier you. Congratulations! I'm so excited to show you how micro changes to your lifestyle will improve your gut health, give you more energy and help you lose weight.

This 30-Day Diet isn't about cutting out food groups or banishing your favourite treats. It's about adding nutritious food to your meals every day to enhance your life and aid weight loss. Say goodbye to food restrictions and hello to incorporating healthier options that nourish your body, aid digestion, improve immunity, and energise your day.

Our motto is simple: empower yourself with every meal. Ready to take those micro steps together? Let's dive in and start improving your life for the better!

THE MAGIC OF THE 30-DAY DIET

The 30-Day Diet will help you harness the power of your microbiome by creating an environment that will nurture and promote good gut health. When I say 'gut', I am referring to your entire gastrointestinal system (GI), starting from the mouth and moving through to the oesophagus, stomach, small intestine and large intestine, and finishing at the lower tract.

In recent years, scientific research has highlighted the crucial role the gut plays in many aspects of our health, including our emotional health and wellbeing. Your gut is your body's main communication system, and it is home to trillions of bacteria, viruses and tiny organisms, known as your microbiome. These organisms send messages to other parts of your body, and shape your health, immune system, happiness and even your weight.

Consider your microbiome as your own personal 'pharmacy' within your body, creating, dispensing and synthesising important compounds like neurotransmitters, vitamins, hormones and enzymes. This pharmacy needs to be nourished with a variety of different foods in order to thrive.

The 30-Day Diet is designed to provide your microbiome with an array of nourishing foods that promote gut health and support weight management.

We're still only at the tip of the iceberg when it comes to fully understanding the complexity of the gut. But we do know it thrives on diversity, so it's crucial we include lots of different whole foods, fresh vegetables, fruits and fermented foods in our diets to ensure we create a vibrant, healthy environment so our microbiomes can flourish.

Why are plant proteins important for gut health?

Plant proteins are found in a variety of foods, including legumes, nuts, seeds, grains and vegetables. They're rich in dietary fibre, which plays a crucial role in maintaining a healthy gut. Additionally, plant proteins are generally easier to digest compared to animal proteins, as they contain less saturated fat and cholesterol. Here are some examples of plant proteins:

- **Lentils:** Not only are these tiny legumes a great source of plant protein, but they are also packed with fibre.
- **Quinoa:** This versatile grain is high in protein and contains all nine essential amino acids.
- **Chickpeas:** Hummus-lovers rejoice! Chickpeas are a fantastic (and delicious) source of plant protein.
- **Garden peas:** Don't let their small size fool you – garden peas are packed with protein and other essential nutrients.
- **Edamame beans:** These young soy beans make a tasty snack and are a great source of plant protein.

FOLLOW YOUR GUT!

Hippocrates, the ancient Greek physician who lived in around 460–370 BCE, famously said: 'All disease begins in the gut.' Referred to as the 'Father of Medicine', Hippocrates believed the key to health lay in achieving balance within the body, as well as lifestyle factors. He saw diet and a healthy gut as essential to overall wellness.

Fast-forward to today, and modern science can support his early insights. We now know the gut's flora significantly affects everything from immune function to mental health, echoing his ancient wisdom that maintaining digestive health is central to preventing disease.

Your gut microbiome is as unique as your fingerprint. It is influenced by your diet, lifestyle, environment, and even how you were born. Comprising bacteria, viruses, fungi and other microorganisms living in your digestive system, this internal ecosystem plays a pivotal role in your health. By understanding and caring for it, you're investing in your overall health, happiness, and longevity. Take care of it, and it will undoubtedly take care of you. Following our plan will help you to regain a happy balance in your gut flora, strengthen your immune system, feel energised and reach a healthier weight.

Digestion and the gut

One of the primary roles of your gut microbiome is to assist in digestion. Your gut helps break down foods, making it easier for your body to absorb nutrients.

The journey of digestion begins as soon as you take a bite of food. Enzymes in your saliva start the process, but it is in the gut where the real magic happens. The microbiome in your gut produces enzymes and chemicals that extract nutrients from food to fuel your body's vital functions.

When your microbiome is in balance, all this happens without a hitch and your digestive system hums along nicely. Nutrients are absorbed, hormones are created, and food travels along at a healthy pace. We may all occasionally experience an imbalance in our gut flora, and suffer symptoms such as bloating, constipation, diarrhoea and even IBS. When this happens, we can be sure there's an internal imbalance in our microbiome.

The immune system and the gut

About 70 per cent of your immune system resides in your gut. This makes sense when you imagine everything you eat and drink has to be scrutinised and checked for pathogens or diseases. Your microbiome has to be able to distinguish between friend and foe, preventing your immune system from attacking your own cells or harmless substances. This function is crucial for fending off infections and keeping your health in peak condition.

Mood and the gut

The gut is often referred to as the second brain. This gut–brain connection can affect our emotions, mood, happiness, eating habits and stress levels. Ever felt butterflies in your stomach when you're nervous? That's your gut–brain connection in action. When we feel stressed, the brain sends signals to the gut through the nervous system, releasing stress hormones. These stress hormones, adrenaline and cortisol, can lead to changes in gut bacteria, potentially affecting digestion and overall gut health.

Chronic stress can lead to weight gain, especially deep in the abdomen area. While it's virtually impossible to eliminate stress from our lives (and the ability to feel stress or fear plays a crucial role in our survival), we do need to manage it better.

Metabolism and the gut

Research shows a strong link between the gut microbiome and metabolism – how our bodies convert food into energy. Certain bacteria types can affect how the body burns calories, stores fat, balances glucose levels and responds to hunger hormones.

By nurturing your gut microbiome with diverse foods, you can create an environment which bolsters and strengthens your metabolism. By eating a more plant-based diet rich in fruits, vegetables, wholegrains and fermented foods like yogurt and kimchi, you'll provide the prebiotics and probiotics your gut loves.

3 micro changes for dealing with stress

Limit stressors – Identify what's causing you to feel stressed. Can you delegate or ask for help? Maybe you need to set boundaries in your life professionally and personally. Unplug from digital distractions, power down your phone, pause your emails, turn off the news and set aside some 'me' time.

Prioritise sleep – Lack of sleep can trigger a domino effect in your body, amplifying stress-hormone production, disrupting hunger signals, and causing mood swings. Make sleep a priority and aim to have seven to nine hours of restorative sleep per night.

Breath mindfully – Breathing might seem automatic, but when we are under stress, our breaths become rapid and shallow. A simple way to change this and reduce stress is to breathe slowly and more consciously. Try it the next time stress creeps up on you, and feel the immediate calm that follows.

THE POWER OF 30

Food scientists now recommend we eat at least 30 different plant-based foods per week to help our microbiome to thrive, to boost immunity and to protect our bodies from inflammation.

Thirty different plant-based foods may seem daunting, but each food brings unique benefits, from fostering beneficial bacteria to reducing inflammation.

Here's a sample of different plant-based foods* to include in your week – it's easier than you think when we show you how. *There are many more plant-based foods – these are just some examples.*

The importance of fibre

When it comes to a healthy diet, fibre is the unsung hero. It may not get as much attention as protein or vitamins, but it plays a crucial role in keeping our bodies happy and healthy. Fibre acts as a prebiotic, providing nourishment for the beneficial bacteria in the gut that help break down food, absorb nutrients and support a strong immune system. Additionally, fibre is a type of carbohydrate that our bodies can't fully digest; as it passes through the digestive system, it helps to keep things moving smoothly. This not only prevents constipation, but also supports a healthy gut.

Which foods are best for fibre?

There are two types of fibre – soluble and insoluble – and it's important to include both in your diets.

Sources of soluble fibre include:
- oats
- nuts
- seeds
- beans
- fruits like apples and oranges

These foods form a gel-like substance in the digestive system, which helps to regulate blood sugar and lower cholesterol levels.

Sources of insoluble fibre include:
- wholegrains
- vegetables like broccoli and carrots
- fruits with edible seeds, like strawberries and kiwis

Insoluble fibre adds bulk to our stools and helps with regular bowel movements.

Good-gut foods

Almonds	rich in fibre, healthy fats and prebiotics	help feed good bacteria
Apples	high in pectin, a prebiotic fibre	support good bacteria growth
Artichokes	packed with inulin, a strong prebiotic	
Asparagus	another excellent source of inulin	supports beneficial bacteria
Bananas	provide vitamins, minerals and resistant starch	promote gut health
Barley	a wholegrain rich in beta-glucan	known to promote healthy gut bacteria
Blueberries	contain antioxidants and fibre	foster a healthy gut
Broccoli	provides dietary fibre and is rich in sulforaphane	may protect gut lining
Brussels sprouts	high in fibre	can prevent constipation and help to foster a healthy gut flora
Carrots	provide fibre and beta-carotene	promote digestive health
Chia seeds	a source of fibre	promote bowel regularity
Chickpeas	fibre-rich	excellent for feeding healthy gut bacteria
Dark chocolate	contains flavonoids	can improve gut flora and reduce inflammation (choose varieties with at least 70 per cent cocoa solids)
Flaxseed	rich in fibre and omega-3 fatty acids	help maintain the gut barrier
Garlic	acts as a prebiotic	helps with the growth of beneficial bacteria
Ginger		helps with digestion and can reduce bloating
Garden peas	packed with soluble and insoluble fibre	
Kale	loaded with fibre and antioxidants	supports overall gut health
Kefir	a fermented dairy drink containing probiotic	can help improve gut flora balance and promote digestive health
Kimchi	a traditional Korean dish of fermented vegetables packed with probiotics	supports gut health and enhance immune function
Kiwi fruit	high in fibre and vitamin C,	helps maintain the lining of the gut
Kombucha	a fermented tea drink containing probiotics and antioxidants	can improve gut health and digestion
Lentils	provide fibre and protein	support gut health
Miso	a fermented soy bean paste rich in probiotics	promotes the growth of beneficial gut bacteria and supports digestion
Oats	full of beta-glucan fibre	beneficial for gut bacteria
Olives	rich in unsaturated fats and high in polyphenols	help foster good bacteria
Onions	high in inulin and flavonoids	promote a healthy gut flora
Pears	high in soluble and insoluble fibre	help with digestion

Pickles	fermented vegetables rich in probiotics	aiding digestion and contributing to a healthy gut microbiome
Quinoa	full of fibre and a complete protein	it has all nine amino acids our bodies need to get from food
Raspberries	high in fibre and antioxidants	packed with vitamin C and antioxidants to lower inflammation
Red grapes	contain the powerful antioxidant resveratrol, especially in the skin	increase microbiome and can help reduce cholesterol and bile acids
Sauerkraut	fermented cabbage rich in probiotics	aids gut health and digestion
Soy beans	high in protein and beneficial isoflavones	
Sweet potatoes	high in dietary fibres	promote healthy gut bacteria
Turmeric	anti-inflammatory	can help reduce inflammation in the gut
Walnuts	high in omega-3 fatty acids and fibre	beneficial for gut health and overall wellbeing
Watermelon	contains both soluble and insoluble fibre	aiding in digestion and promoting a healthy gut
Wholegrains *e.g. brown rice, whole wheat and quinoa*	provide fibre and nutrients beneficial for gut health	support healthy digestion and reduce cholesterol and blood pressure
Yogurt	rich in probiotics, calcium and protein;	supports gut health and aids digestion.

When counting your 30 foods remember that all herbs and spices also count as plant-based foods.

Each meal is an opportunity to add more gut goodness to your plate. We've included many more gut-loving foods in the 30-Day Diet, so you'll easily hit the magic number of 30.

In general, the key is to focus on eating more fruits, vegetables, beans, legumes and lean proteins. They're packed with essential nutrients and fibre, which keep you fuller for longer and provide sustained energy.

LIMIT THE 'BADDIES'

Now we know all the 'good-gut' foods to include in our day-to-day diet, let's have a look at the foods that can negatively impact both gut health and weight management. Here are some common culprits to avoid or limit:

Ultra-processed foods
Ultra-processed foods often contain added sugars, unhealthy fats, preservatives, and artificial ingredients that can disrupt the balance of gut bacteria and contribute to weight gain. Ultra-processed foods include sugary cereals, sweets, crisps, biscuits and processed meats.

Sugary foods and drinks
Excessive sugar intake can feed harmful gut bacteria, leading to inflammation, digestive issues and weight gain. Sugary beverages like sodas and sweetened juices should be limited.

Artificial sweeteners
While marketed as a low-calorie alternative, artificial sweeteners can disrupt the gut microbiome, increase sugar cravings, and negatively impact metabolism, potentially leading to weight gain.

Processed meats
Foods like sausages, hot dogs and deli meats often contain additives and preservatives that can harm gut health and have been linked to weight gain.

Excessive alcohol
While the occasional drink can be part of life's celebrations, excessive alcohol can disrupt the balance of gut bacteria and can contribute to weight gain. Cheers to moderation!

Antibiotics overload
Antibiotics are a lifesaver, but can sweep away good gut bacteria along with the bad. So use them sparingly, and only when absolutely necessary.

HEALTH, HAPPINESS AND WEIGHT

Scientists have discovered a fascinating connection between gut bacteria and body weight. It turns out that individuals carrying excess weight often have different or less diverse bacteria in their gut compared to those maintaining a healthy weight. This amazing discovery highlights that the gut microbiome, not just genetics, significantly influences weight management.

This area of science is still in its infancy, but we know that some bacteria are more efficient at extracting energy from food, which can contribute to weight gain. Furthermore, the microbiome can affect how dietary fats are absorbed, how fat is stored, and how insulin (the hormone that regulates blood-sugar levels) is regulated. A balanced microbiome may help maintain a healthy weight or aid in weight loss by improving metabolism and reducing inflammation, which is often higher in individuals who are overweight.

One thing is for sure: we cannot change our genetics, but we have the power to change our gut health.

Fat facts

Once considered the 'bad boy' of the world of nutrition, we now know that fats are a necessary addition to maintaining a balanced and healthy diet. They are essential for absorbing vitamins such as A, D, E and K, and are vital for brain health, hormone production and the regulation of body temperature. We've included healthy fats in the 30-Day Diet, keeping an eye on moderation.

Here are some tips for incorporating healthy fats into your diet:

- **Use olive oil for cooking and salad dressings** – We've used olive oil spray for moderation.
- **Eat fatty fish at least twice per week** – Salmon, mackerel, sardines and other fatty fish are loaded with omega-3 fatty acids.
- **Snack on nuts and seeds** – Enjoy them on their own, or add them to salads and yogurt for a healthy fat boost.
- **Incorporate avocados** – Add them to salads, spreads or even smoothies for a great source of healthy fats.

EXERCISE FOR HEALTH, HAPPINESS AND WEIGHT MANAGEMENT

Every move, stretch or breath you take is a step towards a stronger, happier you! Exercise is a cornerstone of good health, not just for the muscles and mind, but also for the gut. Incorporating exercise into your daily routine is one of the most beneficial decisions you can make for your gut health and overall wellness, as it improves metabolism, burns calories and boosts overall health. As well as some cardio exercise, we really recommend that you incorporate some type of resistance training into your week. This will keep your body strong and your muscles active, and will help boost your happy hormones.

So grab your workout gear and weave regular movement into your day. Whether you're a beginner or an experienced athlete, the key is to stay consistent and pick a sport or exercise you truly love!

Four ways exercise benefits gut health

1. Enhances gut bacteria diversity – Regular exercise can increase the variety of beneficial bacteria in the gut. These bacteria are essential for everything from digestion to immune system function.

2. Improves gut-barrier function – Physical activity helps to strengthen the gut barrier, protecting against harmful pathogens and reducing the risk of inflammation and associated diseases.

3. Stimulates healthy bowel movements – Exercise facilitates more regular bowel movements, which help in expelling toxins and preventing constipation.

4. Reduces stress – Exercise reduces stress by lowering stress hormones like cortisol, which, when elevated, can harm gut health and alter the balance of gut bacteria when elevated.

Here's how to add some micro movements into your day!

For beginners

Walking
Not only is it free, but it's also easy on your body! Let's get you outside, soaking up some sunshine, boosting your vitamin D, and firing up those endorphins. Commit to a brisk 30-minute walk five days a week, and watch the magic happen.

Yoga
From stressed to zen in no time! Yoga is a fantastic stress-buster that can greatly improve digestion and positively affect gut health. Stretch, strengthen and relax – all in one go!

Cycling
Pedal your way to a fitter you with this fun, low-impact exercise. Whether you're on a stationary bike or exploring outdoors, cycling ramps up your heart health without overloading your joints. Perfect for every age and fitness level.

Take it up a notch!

Jogging
Ready to kick it up a notch? Transition from walking to jogging to boost your cardiovascular fitness even more. It's efficient, ramps up the intensity, and really works those muscles. It's a natural mood-booster, too, releasing happy hormones that make you feel amazing.

Swimming
Dive into this full-body exercise, which is gentle and fun, and a brilliant way to switch off and unwind. Swimming also improves muscle tone and endurance while reducing stress, making it great for your gut microbiome.

Resistance training
Resistance training or strength training isn't just about building muscle and sculpting a toned physique; it also packs a punch when it comes to benefiting your gut health. It can rev up your metabolism, benefit your microbiome, strengthen your core and regulate hormones.

More advanced?

High-intensity interval training (HIIT)

This is a dynamic and efficient form of training which involves short bursts of intense exercise alternated with low-intensity recovery periods. Because of its intensity, HIIT is not only effective for promoting physical fitness and weight loss, but is also proven to significantly improve endurance and metabolic health.

Half-marathon running

For those who enjoy long-distance running, preparing for a half-marathon (or a full one!) can be the ultimate challenge, promoting not only gut health but also incredible endurance and mental toughness.

Regardless of the type of exercise you choose, the benefits to your gut and overall health are extensive.

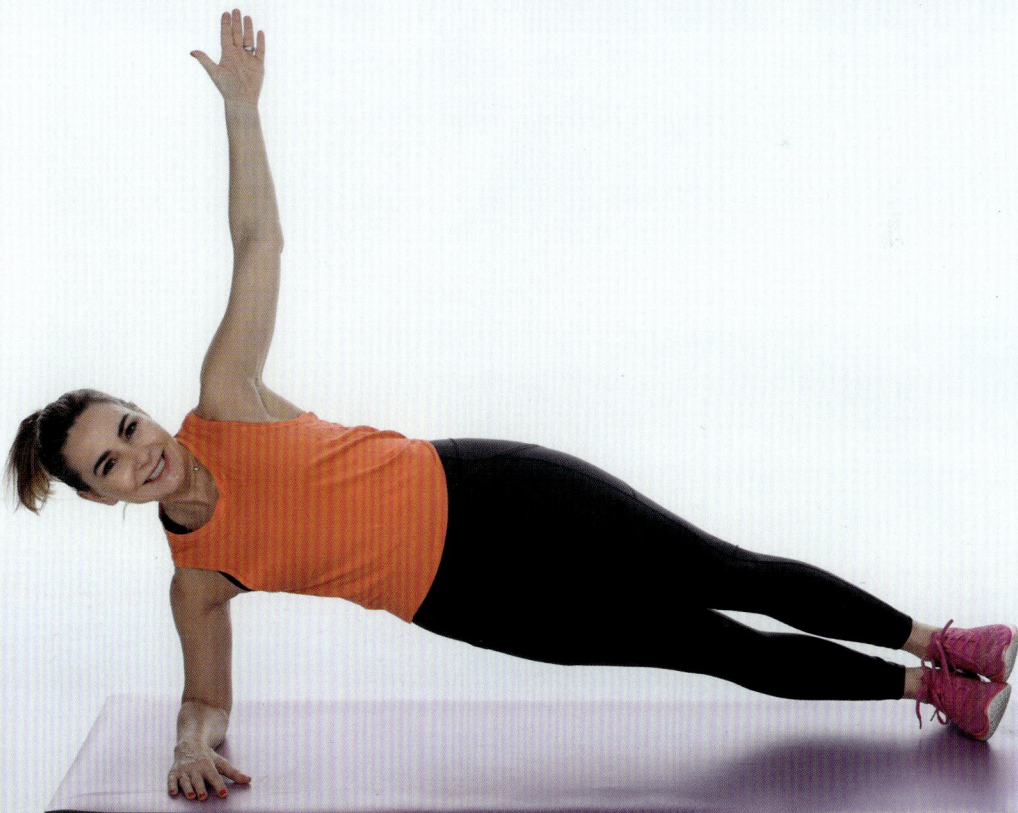

LET'S START THE 30-DAY DIET

The 30-Day Diet is designed to help you rebalance your gut microbiome, energise your body and aid with weight loss. Before you begin this 30-day healthy-eating plan, here's how to get the most out of it.

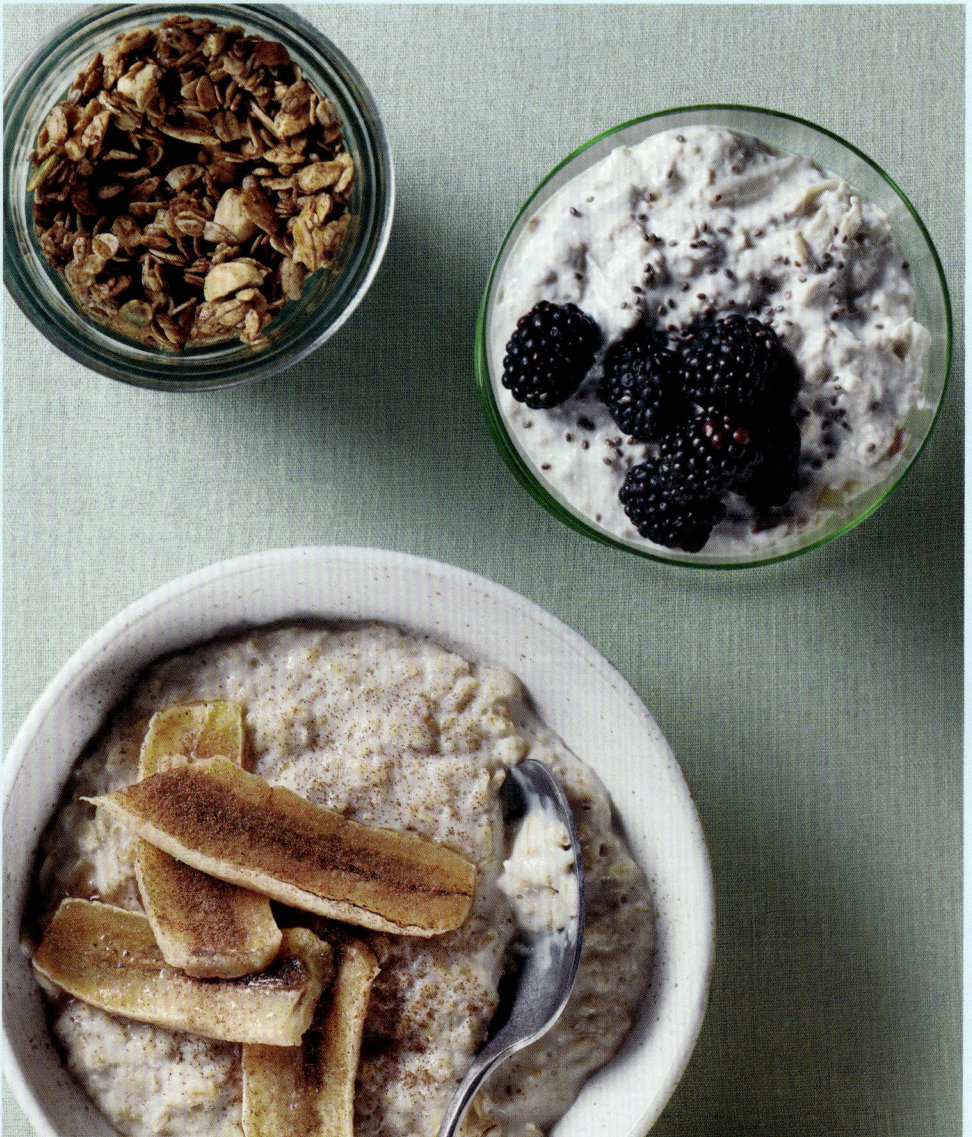

Three plus two

We recommend you eat three healthy meals per day, plus two snacks. This way, your metabolism will remain active, your blood sugars will be balanced and you'll feel energised.

Snacking wisely can be beneficial for your gut health and weight loss. Plan two small healthy snacks a day, one mid-morning and one in the afternoon. As well as keeping your energy up and staving off hunger, healthy snacks can also offer an opportunity to give your body some more gut-loving goodness. Go for something like nuts, seeds, yogurt or fresh fruit (not processed snacks). We've included some tasty snack recipes on pages 103–119, but here are some more ideas you can turn to for a quick and tasty bite.

Greek yogurt with berries
Greek yogurt is rich in probiotics, which are beneficial for gut health, and it's also high in protein, which can aid in weight loss. Adding berries provides antioxidants and fibre.

Almonds and walnuts
Nuts are great for gut health due to their fibre content and healthy fats. Stick to a small handful to keep calories in check.

Carrot and celery sticks with hummus
Hummus is a good source of fibre and protein, and pairing it with raw veggies adds extra fibre and nutrients.

Apple slices with peanut butter
A delicious quick snack that's high in fibre, protein and healthy fats.

Kefir smoothie
Kefir is rich in probiotics. Blend it with fruits like bananas or mixed berries for a refreshing, filling and gut-healthy snack.

Mixed berry salad
Berries are fibre-rich and loaded with antioxidants, which are great for overall health and can help manage inflammation.

Chia seed pudding
More like a dessert, chia seed pudding is packed with fibre, omega-3 fatty acids and protein. Make a pudding with almond milk and a bit of honey for a delicious fibre-rich snack.

Cottage cheese with pineapple
Cottage cheese is high in protein and low in fat, while pineapple can aid digestion due to the presence of the enzyme bromelain.

Air-popped popcorn
Popcorn can be a great low-calorie snack if made without butter or excessive salt. It's high in fibre, which is good for the gut.

Avocado on wholegrain or sourdough toast
Avocado is full of healthy fats and fibre, making this a satisfying snack.

Portion sizes

All the portion sizes in the 30-Day Diet have been worked out for you, but when it comes to making your own choices we recommend you use our plate method, which helps you visualise what a healthy portion size is.

Half of your plate should be filled with vegetables/fruit or salad, a quarter with lean protein, the last quarter with healthy wholegrain carbohydrates. This rule of thumb is very useful when eating out or making dishes outside of the plan.

Our aim is to make healthy eating effortless for you, so understanding what a healthy portion size looks like will ensure you make lasting lifestyle changes.

Flexi-fast

For three days each week, give your body a total break from food for 14 hours every night – from 7pm to 9am, for example. Flexi-fasting is a super way to give your gut an extended break and to regulate good bacteria, which are essential for you to feel your best and digest food better. This simple exercise will help you sleep better, gives your metabolism and gut time to relax, improves digestion and is proven to reduce your calorie intake.

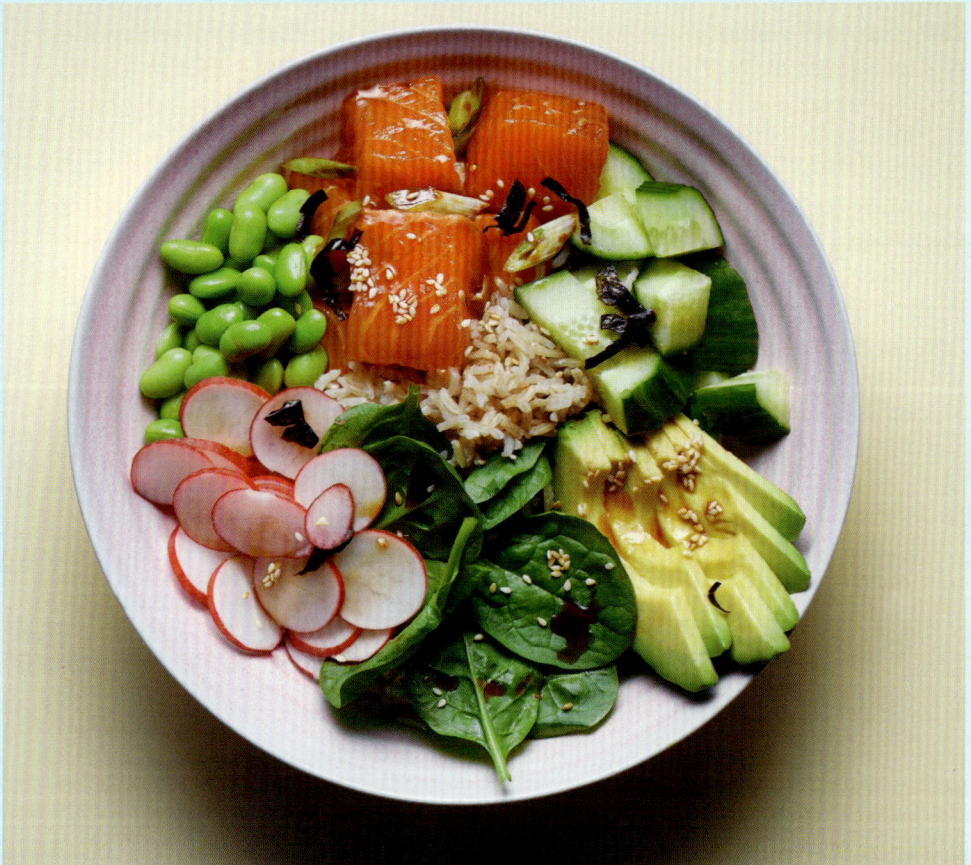

Eating out and takeaways

Eating out or enjoying a takeaway is something most of us do on a regular or semi-regular basis. The 30-Day Diet is a plan for life, so of course you can still indulge in the occasional restaurant meal or takeaway. With a little know-how and some savvy tips, you can enjoy the best of both worlds – satisfying your taste buds while nourishing your gut and maintaining a healthy weight

Preview the menu
Have a look at the menu online and take the pressure off by making your healthy choices before you go.

Don't arrive hungry!
Have one of your healthy snacks before you head out. This way, you won't find yourself filling up on the bread basket.

Make smart swaps
Ask the waiter how the food is cooked, and find out if sauces or dressings can be served on the side. Find out if you can swap fried chips for a side salad or steamed veg. Choose brown rice instead of white, and ask for extra veggies to amp up the nutritional value of your meal.

Choose a salad to start
Ordering a salad before your main meal can help you fill up on gut-healthy, fibre-rich vegetables, which can prevent overeating later. Ask for dressing on the side, and be wary of extras like croutons, cheese and bacon. These can quickly increase the calorie count of your meal.

Order wisely
Opt for dishes that are rich in lean proteins (such as chicken breast, fish or vegetarian proteins like tofu), fibre-packed veggies, and wholesome grains. Look for key words like 'grilled', 'steamed', 'baked' or 'roasted', and steer clear of terms like 'fried', 'battered' or 'creamy'. These foods are often higher in calories and less gut-friendly options.

Be adventurous!
Scan the menu and instead of choosing the obvious, try more plant-based meals which can do wonders for your gut health and waistline. Choose veggie-packed stir-fries, nourishing salads or bean-based dishes to add a fibre boost and support a healthy digestive system.

Watch the portion sizes!
Restaurant portions can be quite large. Consider asking for a half portion, sharing a meal with someone, or setting aside half to take home.

Keep hydrated
Order a jug of water and sip regularly.

Limit high-calorie drinks
Opt for sparkling water or herbal tea instead of sugary drinks, wine or cocktails. If you are drinking alcohol, do so wisely.

Sleep well and start right

Aim for seven to nine hours of quality sleep per night. Lack of sleep can affect the hormones that control hunger and appetite, leading to weight gain. Meditation and sleep hypnosis can help you unwind and get a restful night's sleep.

Set yourself up for success each day by waking up a little earlier, giving yourself time to peacefully enjoy a herbal tea, fill out your journal or watch the sunrise.

Hydration is key

Water boosts metabolism, aids in digestion and helps flush out toxins. Keeping hydrated has so many benefits, including making your skin glow and keeping you energised. Plus, we often mistake thirst for hunger. Remember to stay hydrated by sipping water or herbal tea to support digestion, curb cravings, and help maintain a healthy metabolism.

Mindful eating

Pay attention to what and how you eat. Eat slowly, chew thoroughly and savour your food. Put away your phone, switch off the TV and just enjoy the ritual of eating. This practice helps with digestion and can prevent overeating by giving your body time to recognise when it's full.

Practising mindful eating will help you enjoy your meal more and prevent mindless overeating!

Bon appétit!

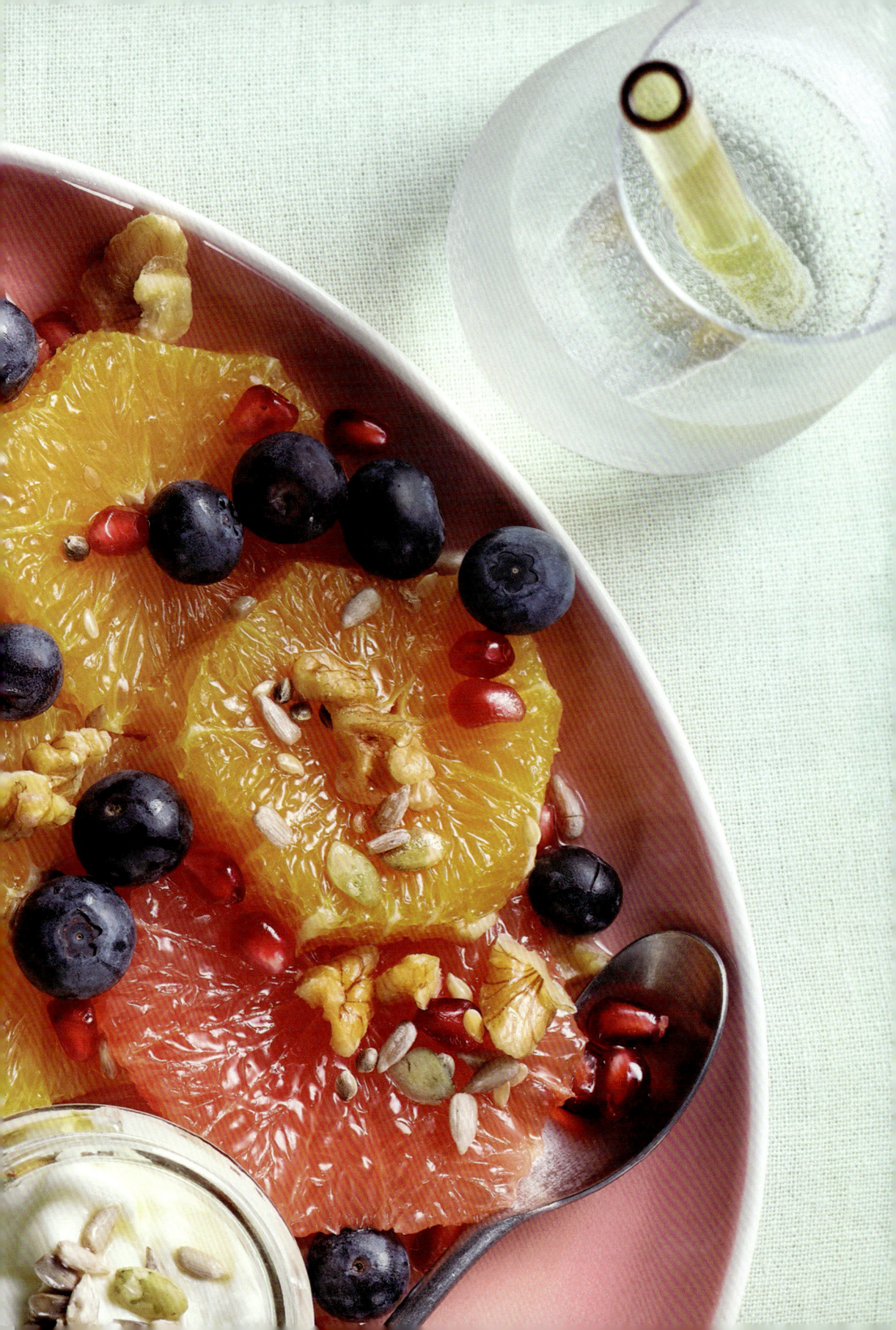

CONTENTS

breakfasts

SPICED PORRIDGE
with cinnamon banana

Starting your day with a bowl of warm porridge is the equivalent of giving your body a nourishing hug. Nutrient-rich and high in fibre, this delicious breakfast offers a slow release of energy and also supports your gut health. We've added a touch of sweetness and extra fibre with a delicious air-fried cinnamon banana. If you don't have an air fryer, you can pop it in the oven or under a hot grill for the same effect (see Note below).

SERVES
1

45g porridge oats
120ml skimmed milk (or unsweetened non–dairy milk)
pinch of ground cinnamon

For the air-fried banana
1 small banana, peeled and halved lengthways
pinch of ground cinnamon
½ tsp caster sugar

PREP
5
minutes

COOK
12–15
minutes

310
kcals
PER SERVING

1. Preheat the air fryer to 190°C.

2. To make the air-fried banana, line the air fryer basket with baking parchment. Place the banana halves in the basket, then dust with cinnamon and sprinkle with sugar. Air–fry for 10–12 minutes, or until the banana is starting to brown and caramelise.

3. Meanwhile, make the porridge. Combine the porridge oats, 120ml water and milk in a non-stick pan and set over a low heat. Stir until the oats start to soften, then increase the heat and bring to the boil, still stirring. Reduce the heat to a low simmer and cook gently for 2–3 minutes until the liquid has been absorbed and the porridge is thick and creamy. Off the heat, stir in the cinnamon.

4. Spoon the porridge into a bowl and top with the banana. Sprinkle more cinnamon over the top and enjoy.

NOTES
If you don't have an air fryer, you can bake the banana in the oven at 200°C (gas mark 6) for 10–15 minutes.

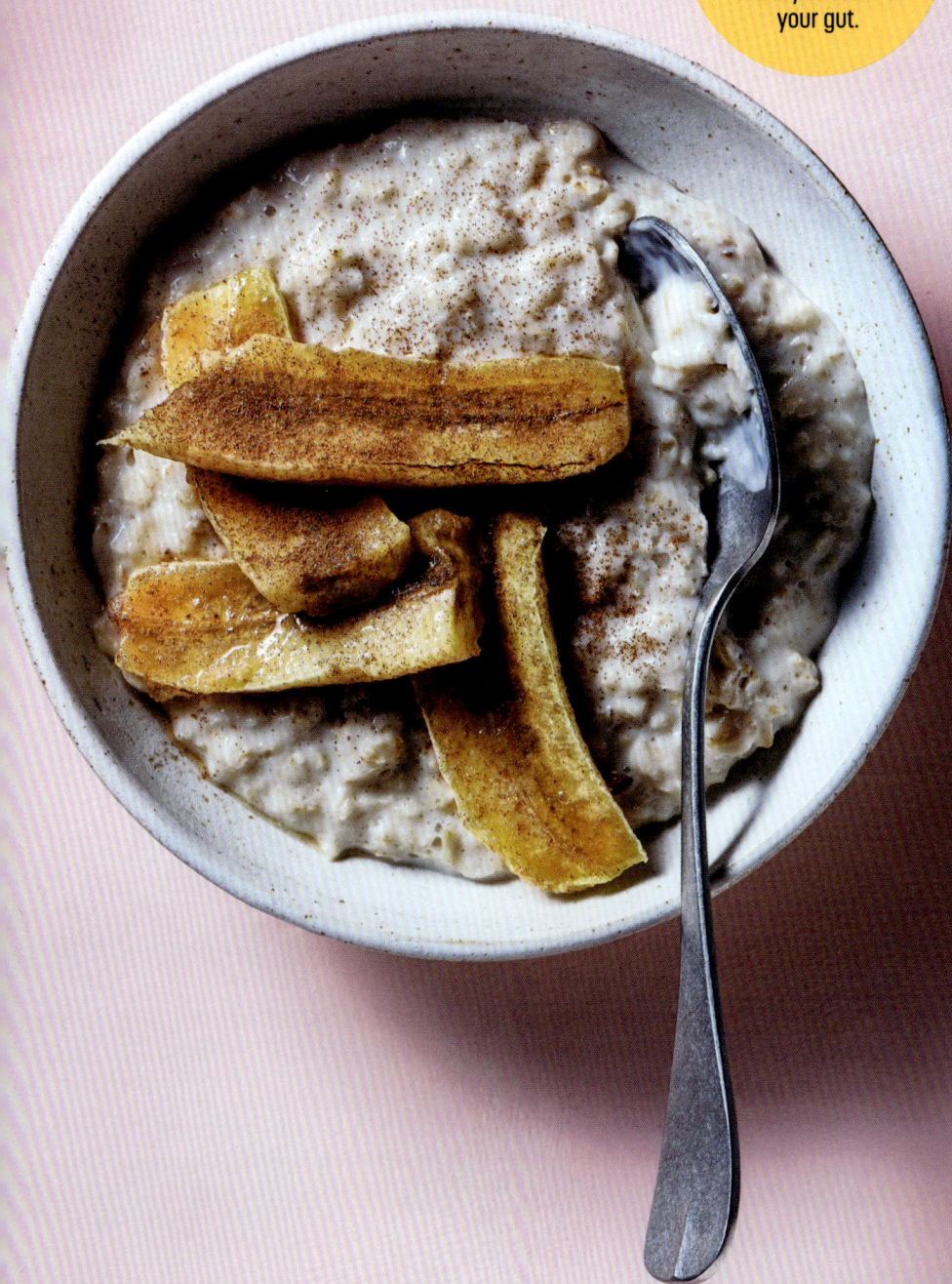

Tip
Top with a spoonful of unsweetened natural yogurt to boost the healthy bacteria in your gut.

FRUITY BIRCHER BOOST

Bircher muesli is full of health benefits and is a delicious way to support your mycobiome, an important part of the gut microbiome. The soaked oats, yogurt and fruit provide fibre, prebiotics and probiotics, which work in synergy to enhance your gut flora. It's easy to make and a great choice for on-the-go breakfasts.

SERVES
2

PREP
10
minutes

SOAK
1
hour or overnight

380
kcals
PER SERVING

4 tbsp unsweetened apple juice
250g fat-free Greek yogurt
1 tsp chia seeds
1 red dessert apple, grated (not peeled)
100g jumbo porridge oats

For the topping
2 tbsp fat-free Greek yogurt
pinch of ground cinnamon, for dusting
100g blackberries
1 tsp chia seeds

1. Whisk together the apple juice and yogurt in a bowl, then stir in the chia seeds, grated apple and oats. Leave in a cool place for at least 1 hour, or overnight, until the oats absorb the yogurt and soften.

2. Divide between two serving bowls and top each bowl with a spoonful of yogurt. Dust with cinnamon, then sprinkle with the blackberries and chia seeds, and enjoy!

Tip
For a good-to-go breakfast, prepare the oats in screw-top jars and chill in the fridge overnight before adding the toppings the following morning. Eat on the way to work or when you arrive.

GOODNESS GRANOLA

Our recipe for low-sugar granola makes four servings, but you can double the quantities and make a bigger batch – it keeps well in an airtight container for a couple of weeks. The oats, nuts, seeds and fruit are packed with fibre, and fermented foods like yogurt and kefir are also good for your gut bacteria. You can vary the fruit and nuts – try rhubarb stewed in orange juice, or some sliced juicy apples and pears.

SERVES
4

PREP
10
minutes

COOK
20–25
minutes

370
kcals
PER SERVING

20g coconut oil (see Tip)
1 tbsp maple syrup or honey
100g rolled oats
2 tbsp chopped hazelnuts
2 tbsp flaked almonds
25g mixed sunflower and
    pumpkin seeds
1 tbsp sesame seeds
1 tsp ground cinnamon

To serve
100g fat-free Greek yogurt
    or kefir
1 small banana, sliced
50g berries, such as
    strawberries, blueberries
    or raspberries

1. Preheat the oven to 170°C (gas mark 3). Line a baking tray with baking parchment.

2. Heat the coconut oil and syrup or honey in a pan set over a low heat. Once the coconut oil has melted, stir in the oats, nuts, seeds and cinnamon until everything is well coated.

3. Tip the mixture on to the lined baking tray and spread out in a thin layer. Bake for 15–20 minutes, stirring once or twice, until golden brown and crisp. Leave to cool before transferring to an airtight container.

4. To serve, spoon a quarter of the granola into a bowl and top with the yogurt or kefir, banana and berries.

Tip
If you don't have coconut oil, use 2 tablespoons vegetable oil instead.

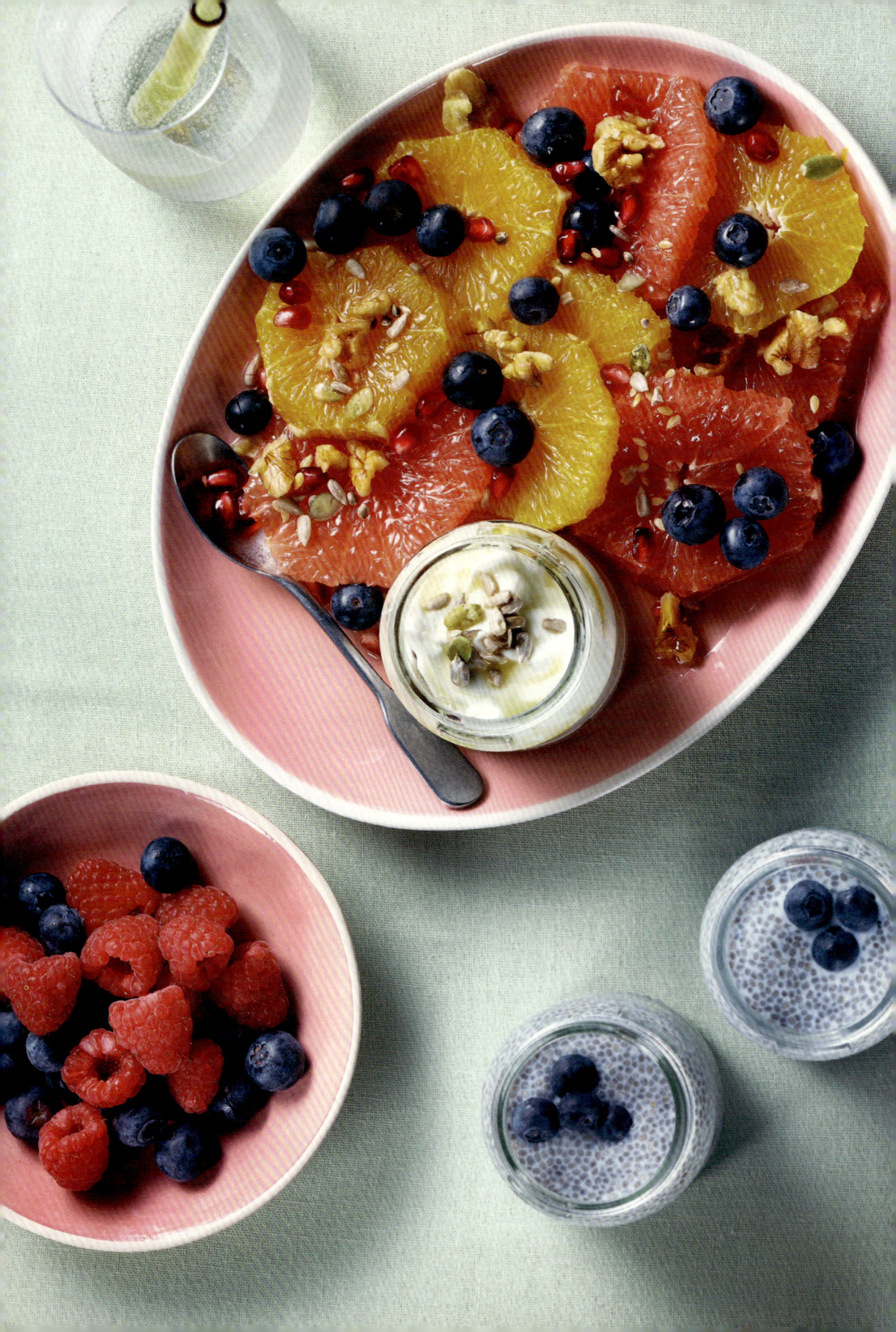

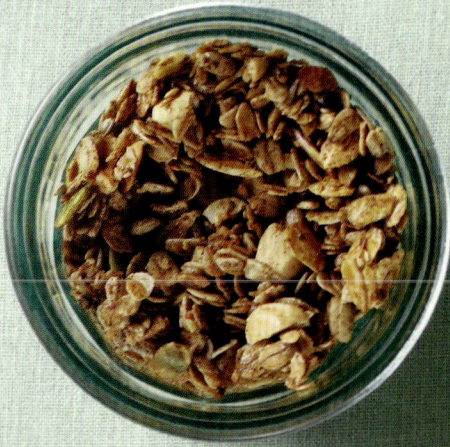

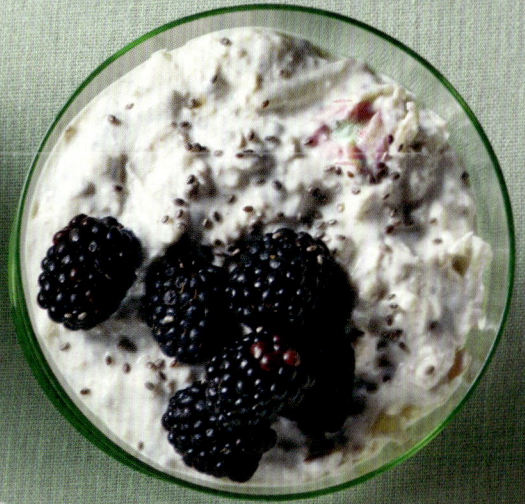

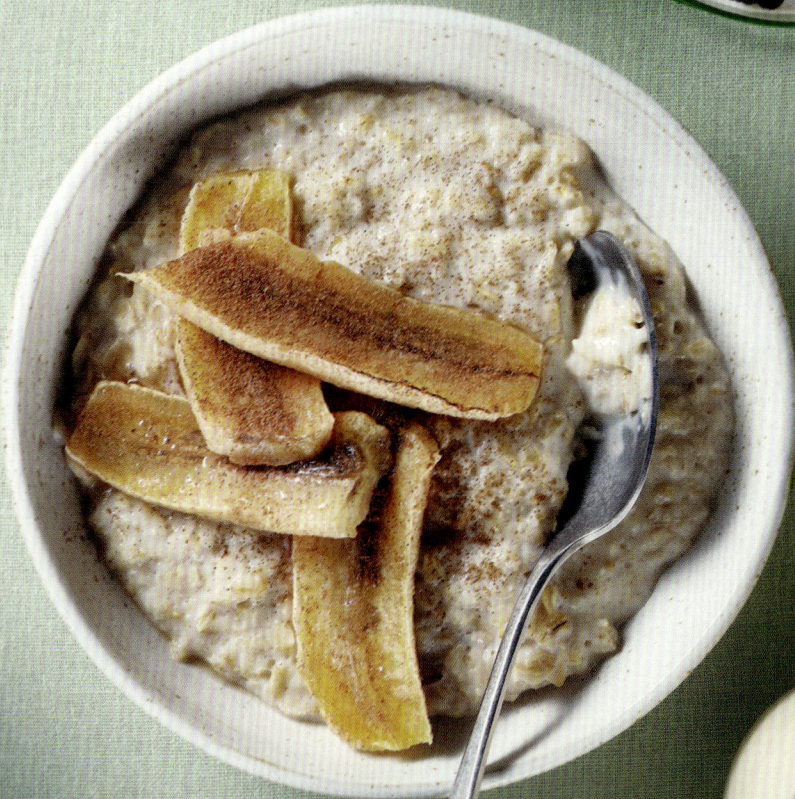

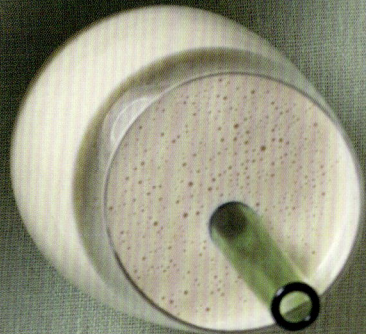

GREEN BREAKFAST OMELETTE

If you love eggs for breakfast but don't have much time to cook, this delicious omelette is for you. It only takes 5 minutes to prep and 5 minutes to cook. You can vary the flavourings: try stirring in some chopped parsley, tarragon or dill, a little diced chilli, or some diced ham.

SERVES
1

PREP
5
minutes

COOK
4–5
minutes

300
kcals
PER SERVING

2 medium free-range eggs
1 spring onion, finely sliced
small handful of baby spinach
    leaves, finely sliced
pinch of ground nutmeg
1 tsp butter or olive oil

25g Cheddar cheese, grated
sea salt and freshly ground
    black pepper
cherry tomatoes on the vine,
    to serve (see tip)

1. Break the eggs into a bowl and whisk. Season with salt and pepper, then stir in the spring onion, spinach and nutmeg.

2. Set a non-stick frying pan over a low–medium heat and add the butter or olive oil. When the pan is hot, pour in the egg mixture, swirling it around to cover the base of then pan. With a wooden spoon, draw the mixture from the side of the pan into the centre so it sets evenly. Sprinkle over the grated cheese.

3. Cook gently for 2 minutes, or until the omelette has set underneath and is just a little runny on top. Sprinkle with the grated cheese, then either flip the whole omelette over to cook on the other side, or fold over one half so you end up with a semi-circle.

4. When the omelette is cooked to your liking and is appetisingly golden brown, slide it out of the pan and serve with cherry tomatoes on the vine.

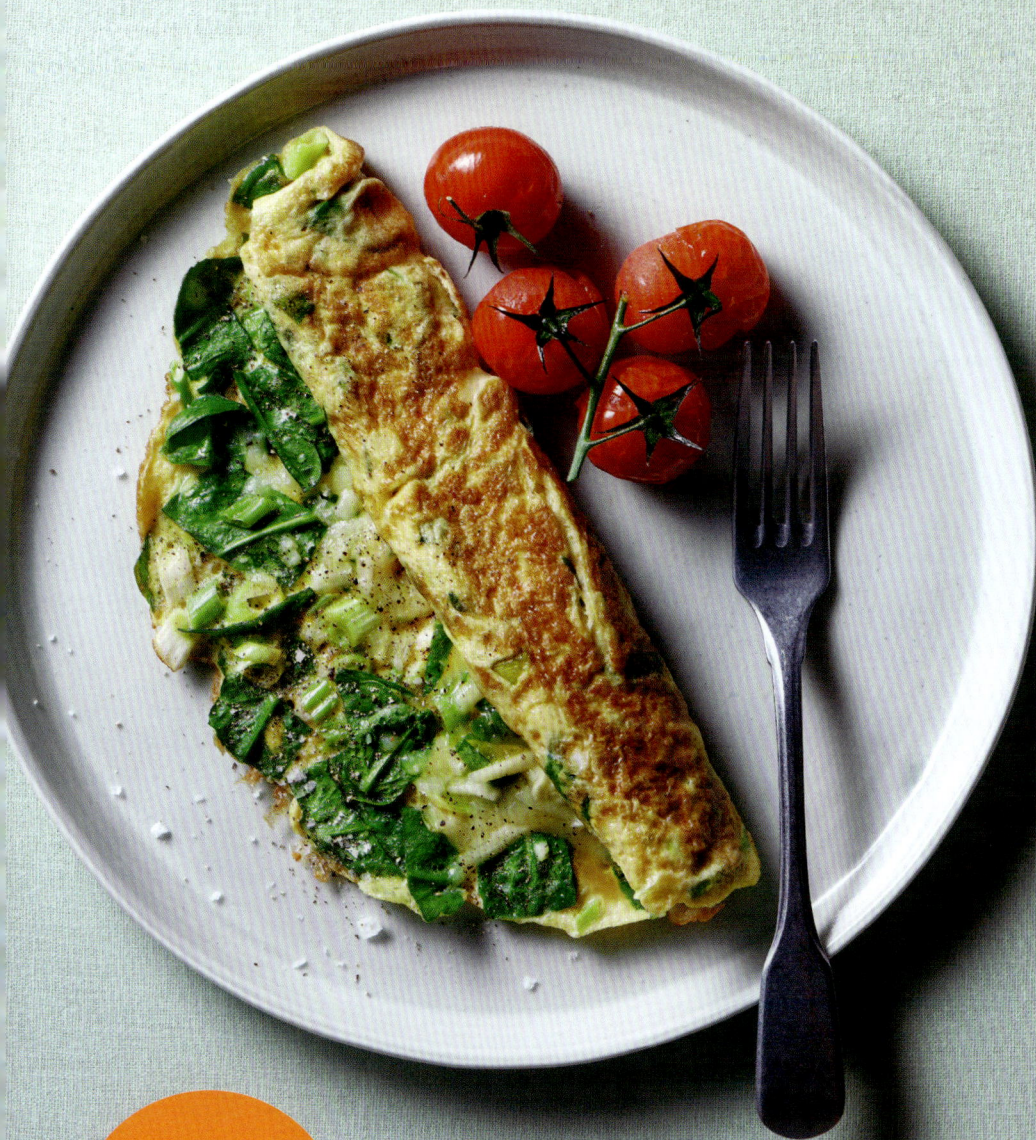

Tip
You can grill or roast the cherry tomatoes, if you wish.

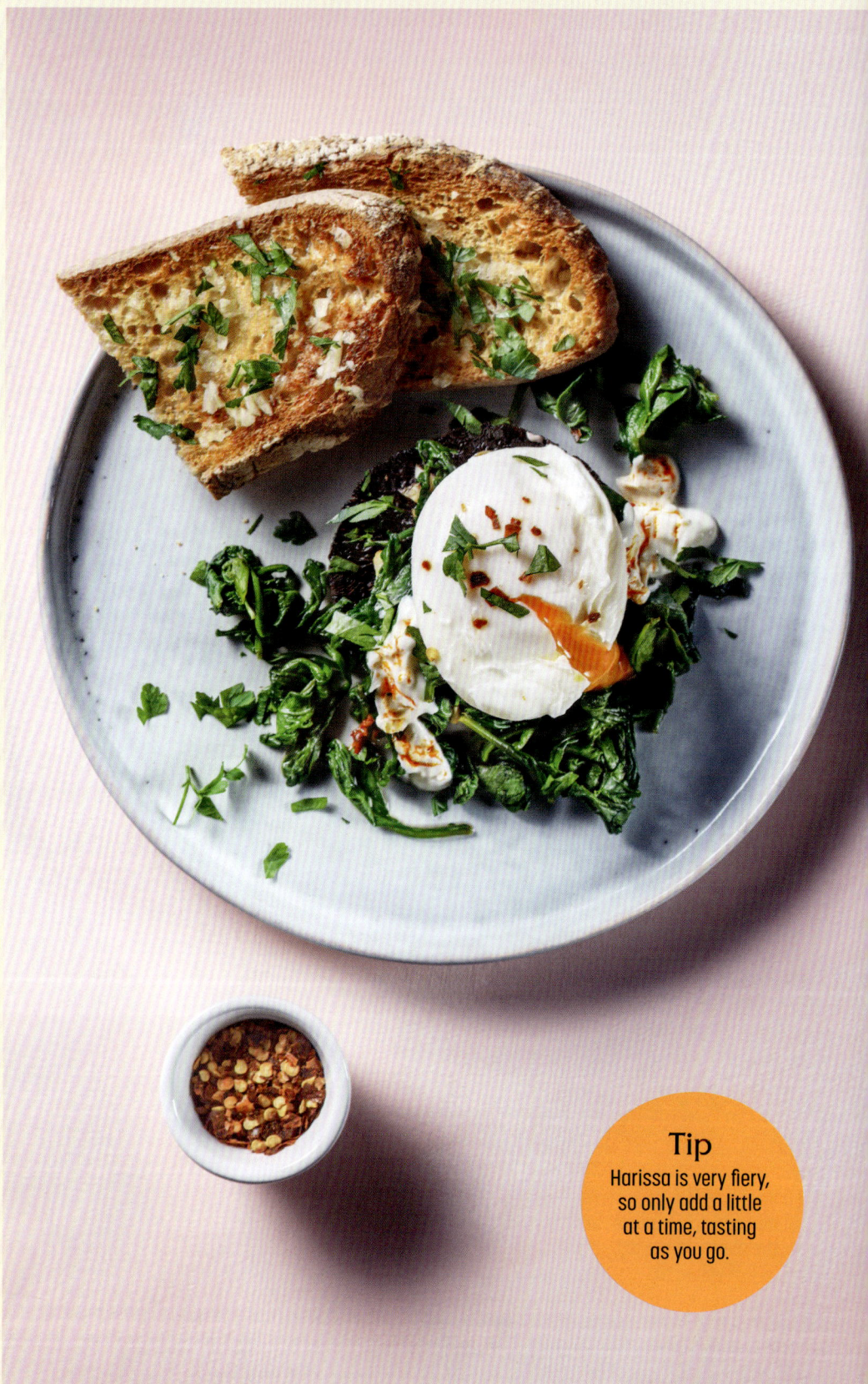

Tip
Harissa is very fiery,
so only add a little
at a time, tasting
as you go.

GREEK POACHED EGGS

Transport your taste buds to sunnier climes with this colourful Greek version of eggs Florentine. With spinach, yogurt, garlicky mushrooms and eggs arranged beautifully on a plate, this is a delicious way to start your day and give your micro-buddies a wake-up call.

SERVES
2

PREP
10
minutes

COOK
5–10
minutes

290
kcals
PER SERVING

200g spinach leaves
1 tbsp white wine vinegar
4 medium free-range eggs
200g fat-free Greek yogurt
grated zest of ½ lemon
½–1 tsp harissa paste (see tip)
pinch of dried chilli flakes
2 slices wholegrain, wholemeal
    or sourdough toast (about
    30g each)

sea salt and freshly ground
    black pepper

For the garlic mushrooms
2 large field or Portobello
    mushrooms
2 garlic cloves, crushed
a few flat-leaf parsley sprigs,
    chopped
olive oil spray

1. Put the spinach into a colander and pour boiled water over the spinach. When it wilts, press down with a saucer to squeeze out the excess liquid. Season with salt and pepper and keep warm.

2. To make the garlic mushrooms, preheat the air fryer to 180°C. Place the mushrooms, gills-side up, in the basket and sprinkle with the garlic and parsley. Spray lightly with oil and season with salt and pepper. Air-fry for 5 minutes. Alternatively, cook under a preheated grill on high for 8–10 minutes.

3. Bring a pan of water to the boil, add the vinegar and reduce the heat to a simmer. One at a time, crack the eggs into a bowl, then slide them carefully into the simmering water. Poach for 3–4 minutes, until the whites are set but the yolks are still runny. Remove and drain on kitchen paper.

4. In another pan, combine the yogurt and lemon zest and warm through on a low heat for 2-3 minutes without the yogurt separating. Season with salt and pepper and swirl in the harissa.

5. Plate the mushrooms and top with the spinach. Drizzle over the yogurt, then top with the poached eggs. Sprinkle with chilli flakes and serve with toast.

ZESTY FRUIT SALAD

This super-fresh, zingy fruit salad is sure to bring a smile to your face. Bright and colourful fruits are like sunshine on your plate, bursting with an array of immune-boosting antioxidants, vitamins and minerals, while energising you for the day ahead.

SERVES
2

PREP
10
minutes

300
kcals
PER SERVING

2 large juicy oranges
1 red grapefruit
80g blueberries
200g fat–free Greek yogurt
1 tsp runny honey (optional)
seeds of ½ pomegranate

2 tsp mixed seeds, such as pumpkin, sunflower and hemp
2 tsp chopped walnuts or pecans

1. Remove the peel and white pith from one orange and the grapefruit. Slice the fruit horizontally into rounds and divide between two serving bowls. Add the blueberries.

2. Juice the remaining orange and pour the juice over the fruit. Divide the yogurt between the bowls and drizzle with the honey (if using).

3. Scatter the pomegranate seeds, mixed seeds and nuts over the top. Serve immediately.

Tip
Instead of the mixed seeds and nuts, top with 2 tablespoons Goodness Granola (see page 33).

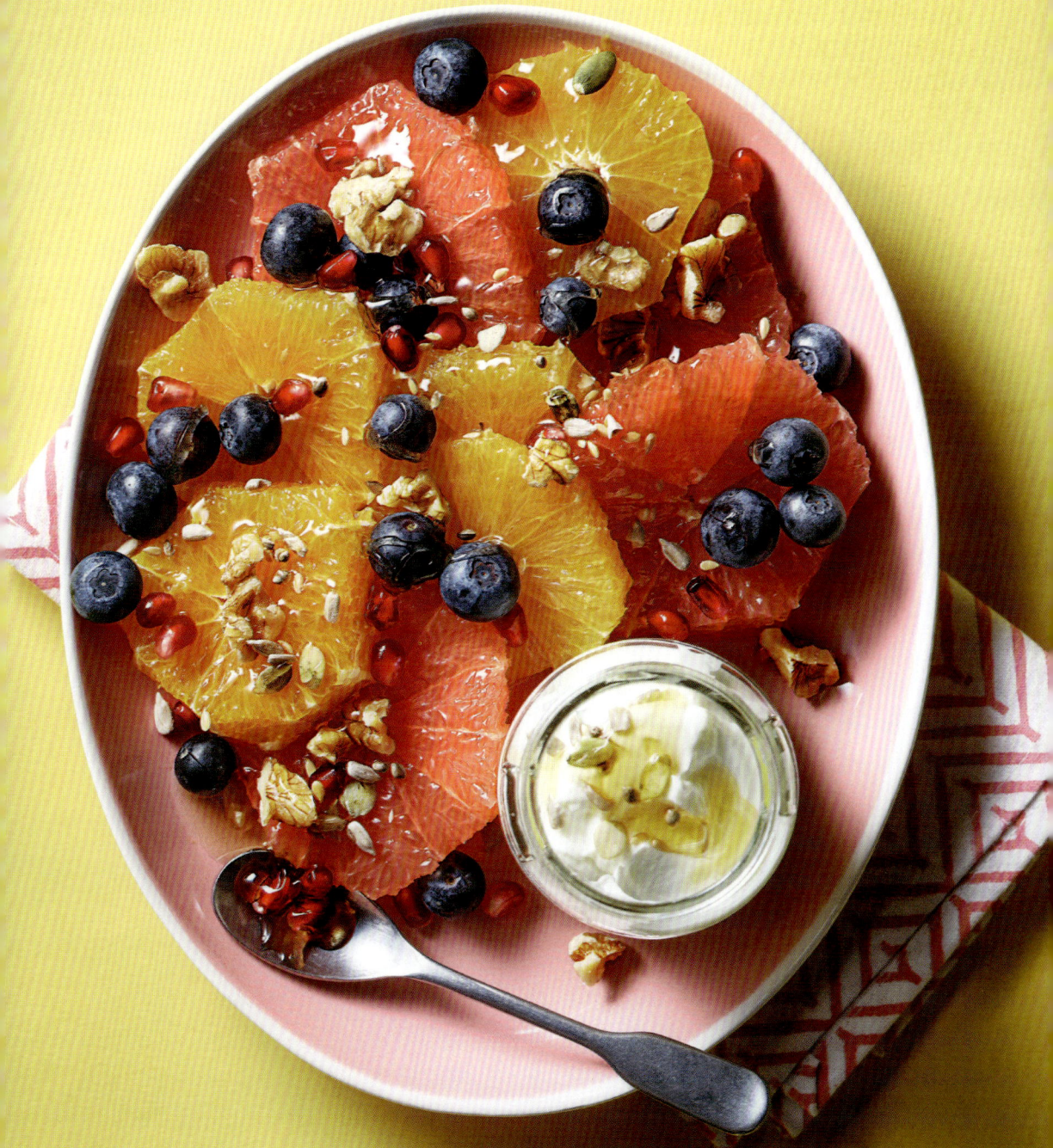

lunches

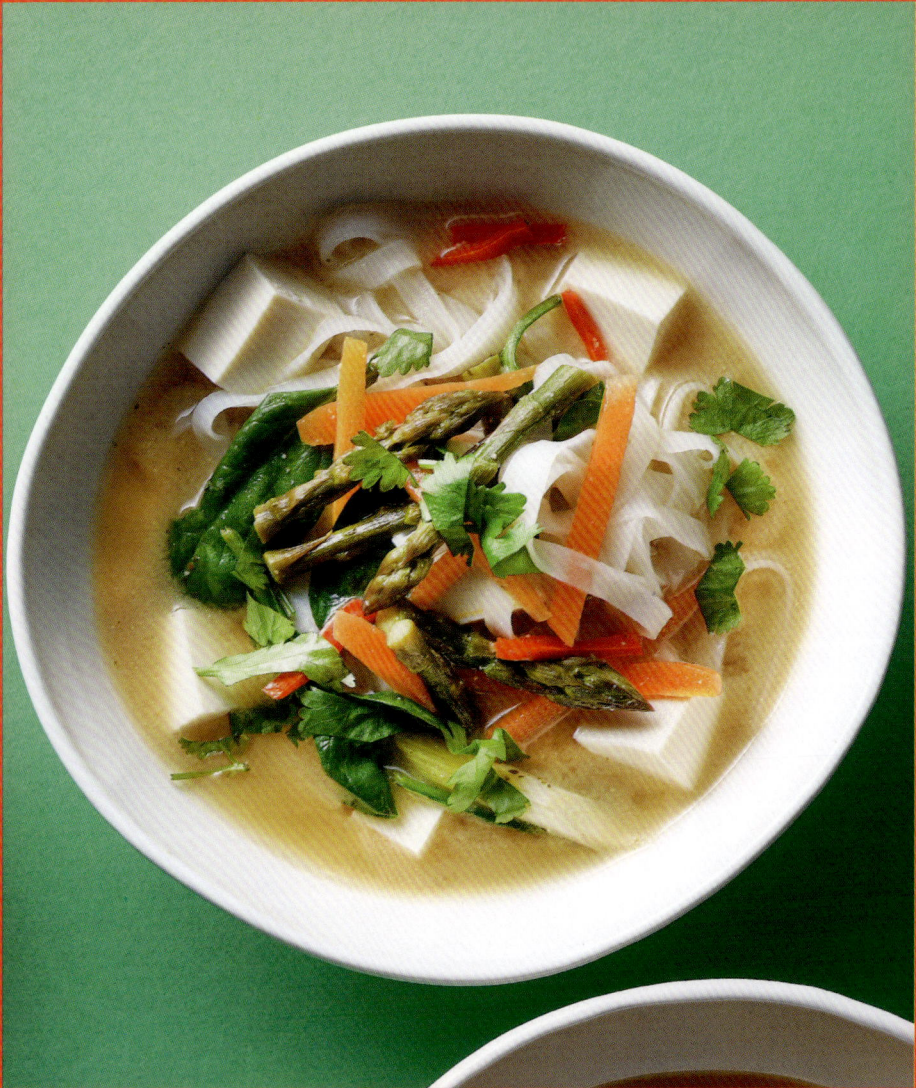

TUSCAN-STYLE BEAN SOUP

This hearty bean soup is full of rich, wholesome flavours that satisfy with every bite. Beans are crammed with powerful proteins and mood-boosting B vitamins. Given the fact that most of your happy hormone serotonin is made in your gut, this bowl of goodness nourishes your microbiome while transmitting feel-good signals to your brain. Good for your gut, good for your life.

SERVES
4

PREP
15
minutes

COOK
1
hour

275
kcals
PER SERVING

olive oil spray
1 large onion, finely chopped
3 celery sticks, diced
3 large carrots, diced
3 garlic cloves, crushed
1 litre hot vegetable stock
400g can chopped tomatoes
2 medium potatoes, peeled and cubed
400g can cannellini or butter beans, rinsed and drained

1 tsp dried oregano
a few thyme and rosemary sprigs
200g Savoy cabbage or curly kale, shredded
handful of flat-leaf parsley, finely chopped
4 tsp green pesto
4 tbsp grated Parmesan cheese
sea salt and freshly ground black pepper

1. Spray a large saucepan with oil and set over a low heat. Add the onion, celery, carrots and garlic, and cook, stirring occasionally, for 8–10 minutes until softened but not coloured.

2. Add the hot stock, tomatoes, potatoes, beans, oregano, thyme and rosemary, and bring to the boil. Reduce the heat to a gentle simmer, then cover the pan and cook for 45 minutes, or until the vegetables are tender.

3. Stir in the cabbage or kale and cook for another 5 minutes, or until the leaves wilt but still retain some bite and look fresh and green. Season to taste with salt and pepper, and stir in the parsley.

4. Ladle the soup into bowls and swirl in the pesto. Serve immediately, sprinkled with Parmesan.

Tip
This soup will keep well in the fridge for up to 5 days. Reheat when you're in the mood for another bowl of happiness.

LUNCHES

BANGKOK-STYLE SIZZLED CORN SOUP

Whipped up in no time, this fiery soup brims with gut-nurturing plant ingredients. It's loaded with fibre-rich sweetcorn, juicy tomatoes, leafy spinach, and anti-inflammatory ginger, all swimming in creamy coconut milk and sprinkled with crunchy nuts. Any leftover soup (spinach and garnishes aside) can be popped in the fridge, where it will stay fresh for up to 4 days.

SERVES
4

PREP
5
minutes

COOK
15
minutes

250
kcals
PER SERVING

2 tbsp Thai red curry paste
400ml can reduced-fat coconut milk
2cm piece of fresh root ginger, peeled and grated
300g canned sweetcorn in water, drained
400g can chopped tomatoes
400ml hot vegetable stock
juice of 1 small lime
handful of baby spinach leaves
1 red bird's-eye chilli, finely sliced
2 tbsp chopped dry roasted peanuts
a few coriander sprigs, chopped

1. Cook the Thai red curry paste in a large saucepan set over a low–medium heat, stirring gently until it releases its oil and starts to sizzle.

2. Add the coconut milk, ginger and sweetcorn kernels, and stir well. Cook gently for 5 minutes, then add the tomatoes and hot stock. Simmer gently for a further 5 minutes, or until heated through.

3. Remove a large spoonful of corn kernels and set aside for the garnish. Blitz the soup, in batches, in a blender or food processor until smooth, then return to the pan. Stir in the lime juice and spinach and check the seasoning.

4. Ladle the soup into four bowls and sprinkle with the reserved corn kernels, along with the chilli, chopped peanuts and coriander. Serve immediately.

Tip
Curry pastes vary in their heat and intensity, so if you prefer mild curry, use only 1 tablespoon and add the rest later.

LUNCHES

CLEANSING TOFU MISO BROTH

Miso broth is utterly delicious, and is renowned for both its umami taste and its gut-healing properties. It's enjoyed by some of the longest-living people in the world, and is an age-old remedy for digestive issues. One bowl will soothe and warm your tummy with an infusion of beneficial pre- and probiotics. To elevate the flavour, use the best-quality vegetable stock you can find, or go one step further by making your own. Simply save leftover vegetable skins, peelings, tops and tails (our faves are carrots, celery and onion), simmer in a pan of water for several hours with fresh herbs and spices, then strain. Delicious!

SERVES
4

PREP
10
minutes

COOK
12–15
minutes

215
kcals
PER SERVING

1 litre hot vegetable stock
4 tbsp white miso paste
8 spring onions, sliced
3 garlic cloves, crushed
2.5cm piece of fresh root ginger, peeled and grated
1 red chilli, deseeded and finely sliced
1 large carrot, cut into thin matchsticks

200g fine asparagus spears, trimmed and sliced
250g spinach leaves, sliced
200g pre-cooked thin rice noodles
225g silken tofu, cubed
dash of lime juice
a few drops of light soy sauce, to taste
handful of coriander, chopped

1. Pour the stock into a large saucepan and bring to the boil. Reduce the heat to a simmer and add the miso paste. Stir with a wooden spoon until it dissolves.

2. Reduce the heat to low and add the spring onions, garlic, ginger, chilli, carrot and asparagus. Simmer gently for 4–5 minutes, then stir in the spinach and rice noodles and cook for a further 3–4 minutes.

3. Add the tofu and lime juice, plus soy sauce to taste, and cook for 1 minute to gently heat through.

4. Stir in the coriander, then ladle the soup into four serving bowls and serve immediately.

Tip
Try adding some l ong-stem broccoli and shiitake mushrooms. The soup will keep well in a sealed container in the fridge for a couple of days.

SPICY BUTTERNUT SQUASH & GINGER SOUP

Ginger, spice and everything nice come together in this heart-warming soup with a gentle kick of chilli, turmeric and fresh ginger. Bright orange butternut squash is rich in antioxidants, which acts as a guardian for your gut lining. All infused with the anti-inflammatory benefits of fresh coconut milk, this soup is a hug for your tummy.

SERVES
4

PREP
20
minutes

COOK
35
minutes

250
kcals
PER SERVING

olive oil spray
1 onion, chopped
3 celery sticks, diced
2 garlic cloves, crushed
2.5cm piece of fresh root ginger, peeled and diced
3 large carrots, chopped
500g butternut squash, peeled, deseeded and diced
600ml hot vegetable stock
300ml canned reduced-fat coconut milk
2 tsp ground turmeric
1 tsp ground cumin
½ tsp ground cinnamon
½ tsp freshly grated nutmeg
handful of parsley, finely chopped
pinch of dried chilli flakes
sea salt and freshly ground black pepper

For the crispy croutons
2 slices of sourdough bread (about 30g each), cut into small cubes
2 tsp olive oil

1. Preheat the oven to 180°C (gas mark 4) and line a baking tray with baking parchment.

2. Tip the bread cubes into a bowl. Add the olive oil and toss until coated. Spread on the prepared tray and bake for 15–20 minutes, turning halfway, until crisp and golden brown.

3. Meanwhile, lightly spray a large saucepan with oil and set over a low–medium heat. Cook the onion, celery, garlic, ginger and carrots for 10 minutes, stirring until tender but not coloured. Add the squash and cook for 5 minutes.

4. Add the hot stock and bring to a simmer for 15 minutes, or until the vegetables are tender.

Tip
You can use pumpkin instead of squash.

5. Working in batches, blitz the soup in a blender or food processor until smooth. Return it to the pan and stir in the coconut milk and spices. Reheat gently, stirring occasionally, over a low heat. Season to taste and stir in the parsley.

6. Divide between four bowls and serve topped with the chilli flakes and crispy croutons.

LUNCHES

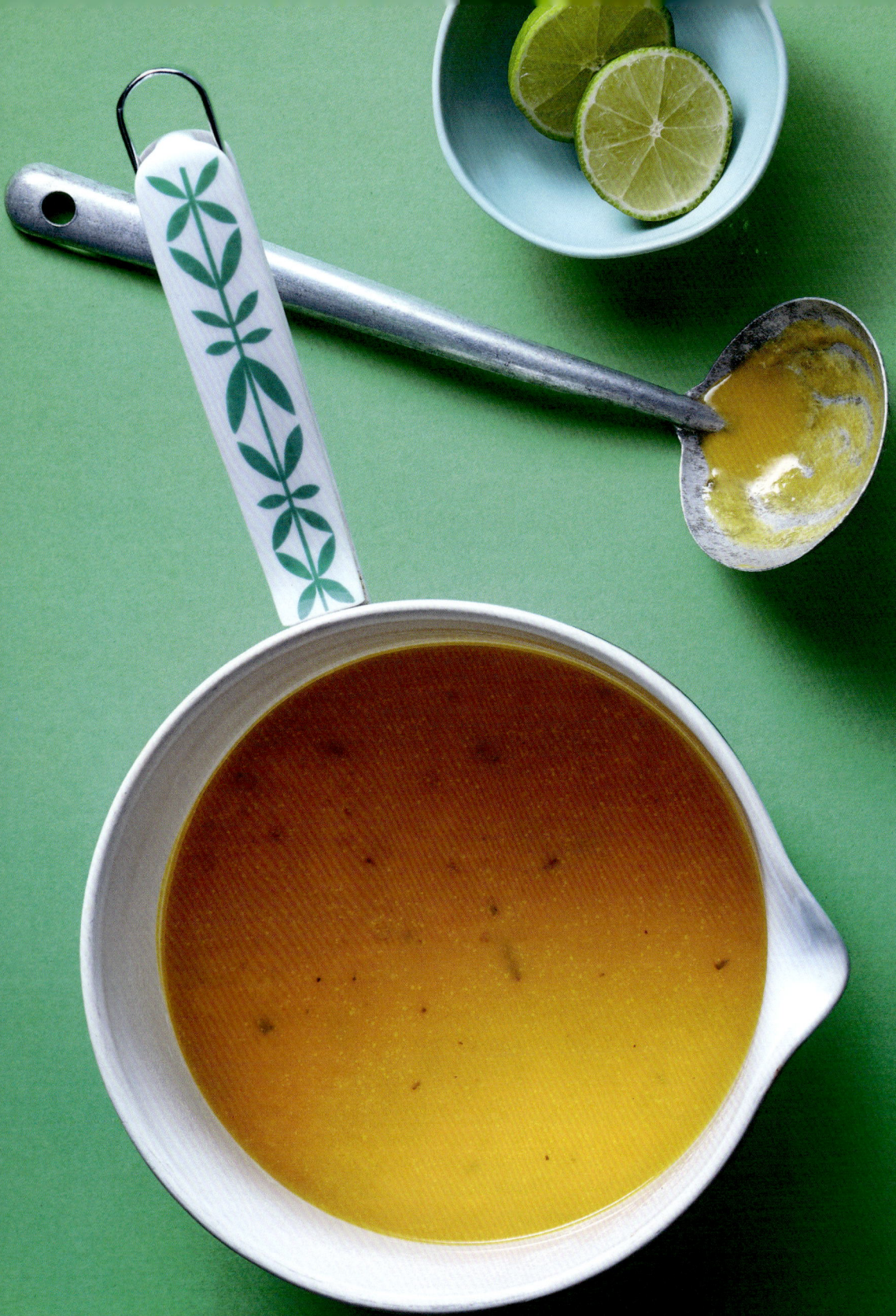

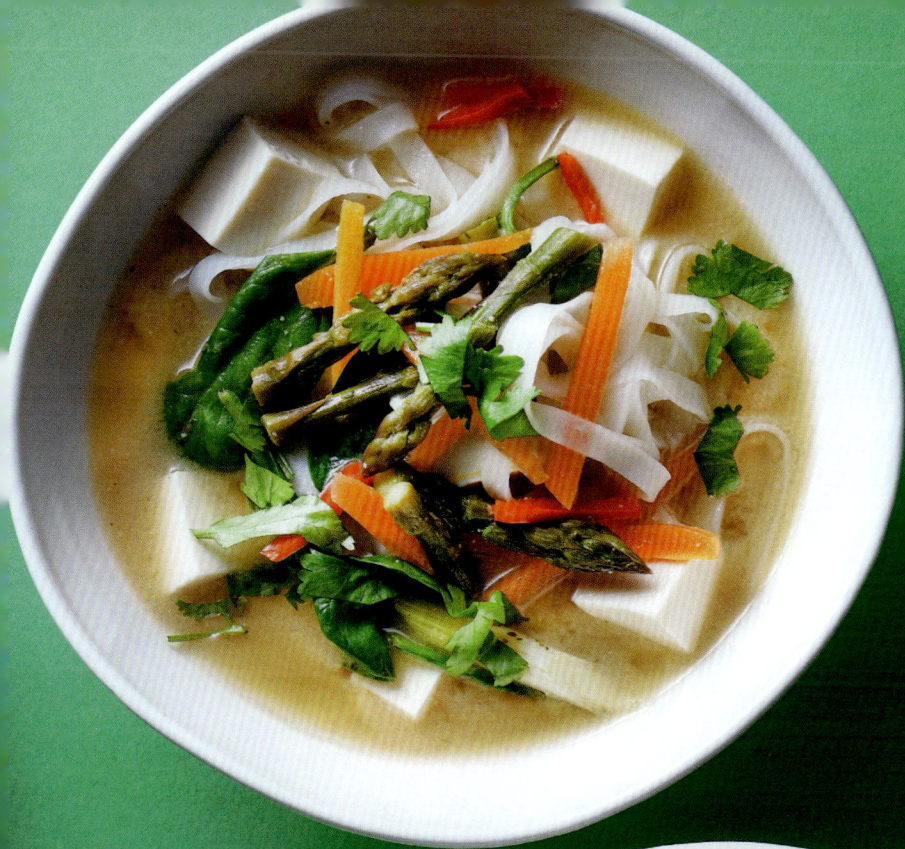

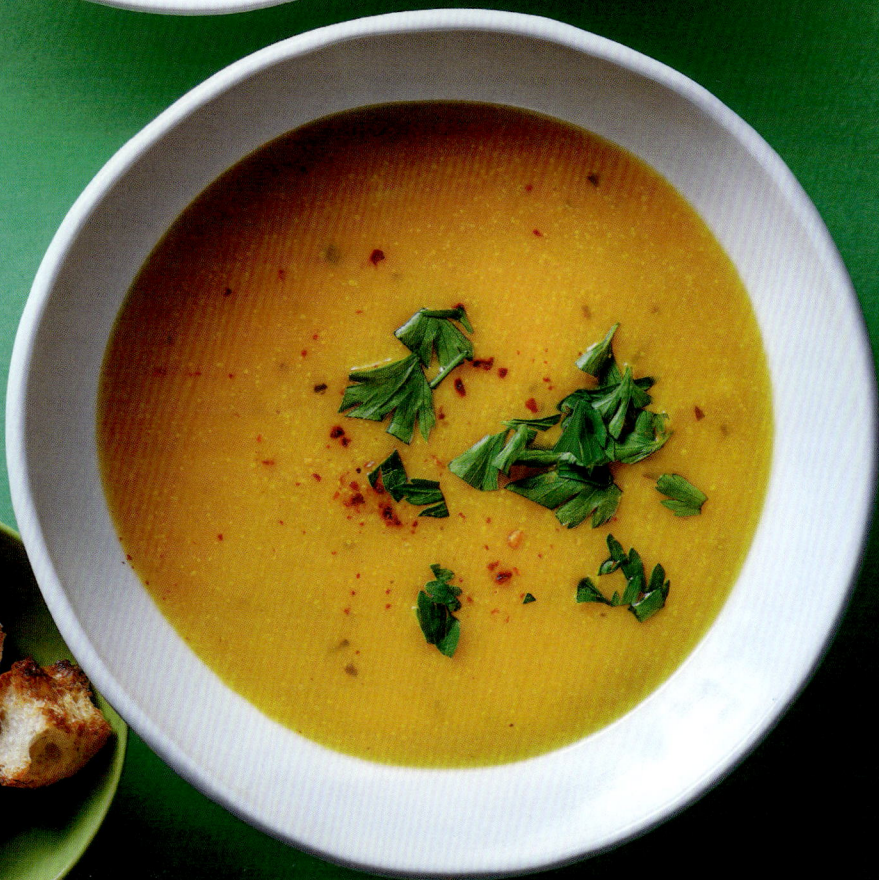

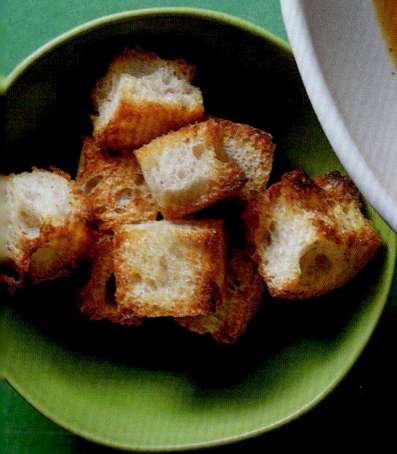

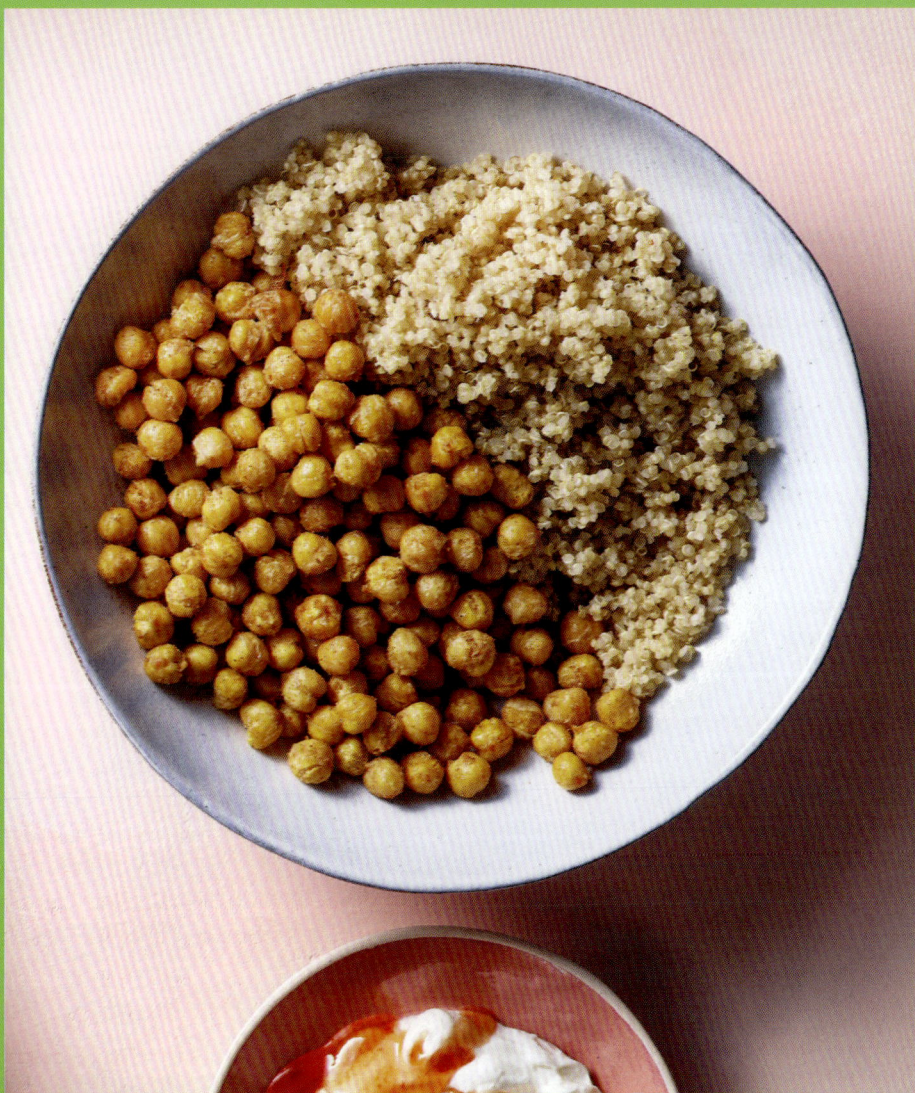

RAINBOW CHOPPED SALAD
with sesame dressing

This vibrant salad is a feast for the eyes and a best friend for your microbiome. Quinoa is a powerhouse when it comes to supporting gut health, while avocado adds a creamy texture and a dose of healthy fats, and the mango provides a sweet contrast and additional vitamins. The flavour-filled dressing, with its blend of sesame oil, lime juice and fish sauce, introduces a tangy depth and health benefits of its own.

SERVES
2

PREP
10
minutes

365
kcals
PER SERVING

1 red pepper, chopped
½ cucumber, diced
¼ red onion, diced
100g sugar snap peas, chopped
1 small avocado, peeled, stoned and diced
100g mango, peeled, stoned and diced
200g peeled cooked prawns

handful of mint leaves, chopped
handful of coriander, chopped
100g cooked quinoa

For the sesame dressing
2 tsp sesame oil
1 tbsp nam pla (Thai fish sauce)
juice of 1 lime
1 tbsp sweet chilli sauce
pinch of sea salt crystals

1. In a large bowl, combine all the chopped vegetables, along with the mango, prawns, herbs and quinoa.

2. In a small bowl, combine all the dressing ingredients and whisk well.

3. Pour the dressing over the salad and toss to coat. Season to taste with salt, then spoon into two bowls and enjoy!

NOTE
If you don't have time to cook the quinoa yourself, you can use a pouch of ready-cooked grains (available in most delis and supermarkets). This is a great way to increase your fibre intake.

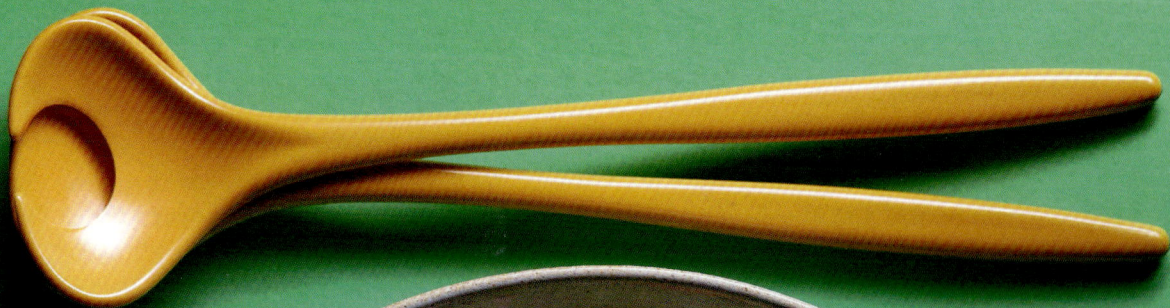

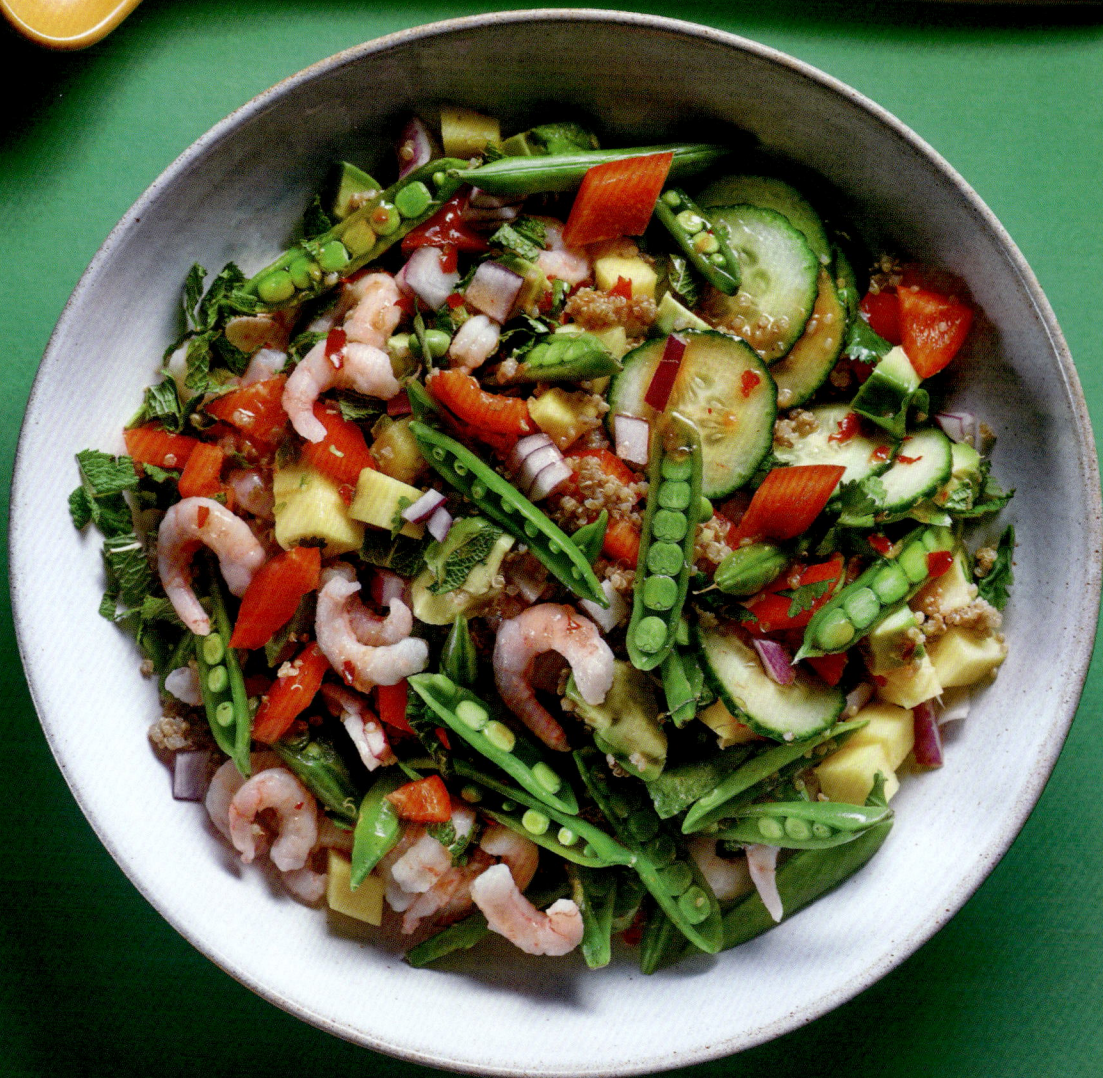

Tip
This salad also tastes delicious with bulghur wheat, brown rice or spelt.

LENTIL & GREENS SALAD JAR

This layered lentil salad jar is the perfect portable lunch for when you're on the go. Powerful proteins and fibre-rich, heart-healthy nutrients are topped off with a creamy tahini dressing. Divine!

SERVES
1

PREP
15
minutes

COOK
20
minutes

390
kcals
PER SERVING

100g sweet potato, peeled and cut into small cubes
olive oil spray
¼ small red onion, diced
3 cherry tomatoes, sliced
75g cooked green or brown lentils (see tip)
handful of curly kale, woody stems removed

30g feta cheese, diced
sea salt and freshly ground black pepper

For the tahini dressing
2 tsp tahini
2 tsp soy sauce
1 tsp maple syrup or runny honey
1 tsp lemon juice

1. Preheat the oven to 190°C (gas mark 5).

2. Spread out the sweet potato cubes on a baking sheet and spray lightly with oil. Season with salt and pepper, and bake in the oven for 20 minutes, or until cooked through and tender.

3. Meanwhile, make the tahini dressing: whisk all the ingredients together in a bowl until smooth. If it's a bit too thick, add a few drops of water or more lemon juice to thin.

4. Pour the dressing into the bottom of a Mason jar. Add a layer of red onion, followed by a layer of tomatoes.

5. Next, add the cooked lentils, followed by the sweet potato cubes. Top with the curly kale and, lastly, the feta. Screw on the lid of the jar.

6. If you're making this salad the day before you plan to eat it, keep in the fridge overnight. Just before serving, shake the Mason jar to distribute the dressing, then transfer the contents into a bowl.

NOTE
When making a salad jar, always put the dressing in first and layer the firmer vegetables at the bottom, the protein in the middle and the softer ingredients and leafy greens at the top.

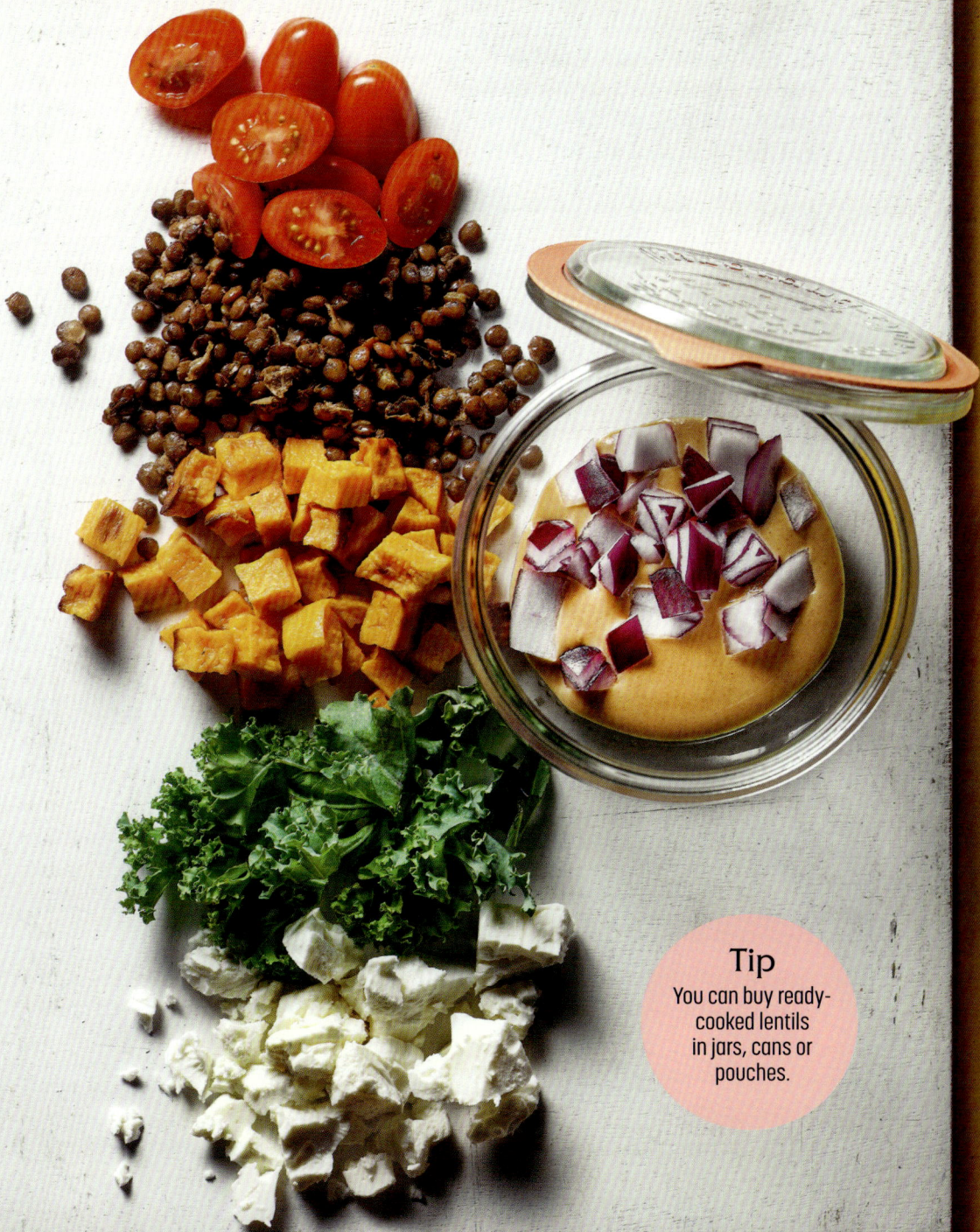

Tip
You can buy ready-cooked lentils in jars, cans or pouches.

CREAMY CHICKEN CAESAR SALAD

Our chicken Caesar salad features a creamy dressing made with fat-free Greek yogurt, which is a gut-loving, muscle-fuelling dollop of goodness! For an extra splash of colour and crunch we've sprinkled in shredded kale, which boosts your digestion and nurtures the growth of beneficial gut bacteria, making every bite not just tasty but also wholesome.

SERVES
2

PREP
15
minutes

COOK
10
minutes

390
kcals
PER SERVING

2 slices of stale wholemeal bread (about 30g each), cut into cubes
olive oil spray
200g skinless chicken breast fillets
1 head cos lettuce, shredded
60g fresh kale, stems removed, shredded
2 tbsp grated Parmesan cheese

For the Caesar dressing
1 garlic clove, crushed
½ tsp Dijon mustard
1 anchovy fillet, rinsed and drained
40g Parmesan cheese, grated
2 tbsp lemon juice
2 tsp olive oil
3 tbsp fat-free Greek yogurt
a few drops of Worcestershire sauce (optional)

1. Preheat the oven to 150°C (gas mark 2).

2. Spread out the bread cubes on a baking tray. Lightly spray with oil and bake in the oven for 10 minutes until you have crisp, golden croutons.

3. Meanwhile, lightly spray a ridged non-stick griddle pan with oil and set over a medium heat. When the pan is hot, add the chicken and cook, turning occasionally, for 8–10 minutes until golden brown and crisp on the outside and cooked right through inside. Cut into cubes.

4. To make the Caesar dressing, blitz the garlic, mustard, anchovy, Parmesan cheese and lemon juice in a blender. Add the oil and yogurt, and blend briefly until combined. Taste and, if wished, add a few drops of Worcestershire sauce.

5. Add the lettuce, kale and croutons to a large bowl. Pour over the dressing and toss to combine, then divide between two serving plates. Scatter the warm chicken over the top and sprinkle with grated Parmesan to serve.

Tip
If you don't like anchovies, just make the dressing without.

THAI-STYLE CAULIFLOWER RICE SALAD with lime dressing

This bright, colourful salad fuses tangy citrus flavours with a salty, sweet, spicy kick. Cauliflower is a superhero in the veggie world and it provides a hefty dose of vitamin K, ensuring your bones stay strong, and it's loaded with vitamin C to help ward off colds.

SERVES
2

PREP
15
minutes

COOK
6–8
minutes

CHILL
15
minutes

250
kcals
PER SERVING

½ small cauliflower, stem removed, separated into florets
olive oil spray
1 lemongrass stalk, peeled and diced
1 red chilli, diced
5 spring onions, finely sliced
75g grated carrot
75g grated courgette
2 cooked skinless chicken breast fillets (about 100g each), shredded

2 lime leaves, finely sliced
handful of mint, finely chopped
handful of coriander, finely chopped

For the lime dressing
juice of 2 limes
1 tbsp nam pla (Thai fish sauce)
1 tsp caster sugar

1. Put the cauliflower florets into a food processor and pulse until they have the consistency of rice.

2. Lightly spray a wok or frying pan with oil and set over a medium–high heat. Add the lemongrass, chilli and spring onions, and stir-fry for 2–3 minutes. Add the cauliflower 'rice' and stir-fry for another 4–5 minutes until just tender.

3. Transfer to a large bowl and stir in the carrot, courgette, chicken, lime leaves and herbs.

4. To make the dressing, stir all the ingredients together in a small bowl until well blended and the sugar has dissolved. Pour over the cauliflower mixture and gently toss

5. Cover with a lid or cling film and chill in the fridge for at least 15 minutes before serving.

Tip
Instead of chicken, you could use cooked peeled prawns, edamame beans or crispy grilled tofu.

NOTE
Easily made in advance, you can pop this into the fridge for several hours or even overnight, making it the perfect choice for packed lunches.

SICILIAN ORANGE & FENNEL SALAD

The dreamy combo of orange and fennel works its magic in this refreshing salad. The sun-drenched flavours of Sicily sing with ruby-red pomegranate seeds, creamy avocado and crumbled feta topping. Every ingredient brings joy to your gut, with fennel being a particular hero when it comes to aiding digestion and reducing inflammation.

SERVES
2

PREP
15
minutes

STAND
15
minutes

420
kcals
PER SERVING

½ red onion, finely sliced
1 tbsp apple cider vinegar
1 medium fennel bulb
2 small juicy oranges
8 black olives, pitted
1 small ripe avocado, peeled, stoned and cubed

seeds of ½ pomegranate
1 tbsp fruity green olive oil
juice of 1 small lemon
pinch of crushed sea salt
100g feta cheese, crumbled
handful of mint, chopped

1. Place the onion slices in a bowl and pour over the vinegar. Set aside while you prepare the other vegetables.

2. Cut the base off the fennel and trim the long stalks on top, removing the feathery fronds. Thinly slice the fennel bulb and place in a large bowl. Chop the stalks and feathery fronds and set aside.

3. Cut the top and base off each orange and remove the outer peel and white pith with a sharp knife. Cut each orange horizontally into slices, then cut each slice into quarters. Add these to the bowl with the fennel, along with any juices.

3. Add the olives, avocado, pomegranate seeds and reserved fennel stalks and fronds to the bowl, then gently stir in the red onion. Drizzle with the olive oil and lemon juice, then sprinkle with salt. Set aside for at least 15 minutes to allow the flavours to develop.

4. Just before serving, scatter the feta and mint over the top.

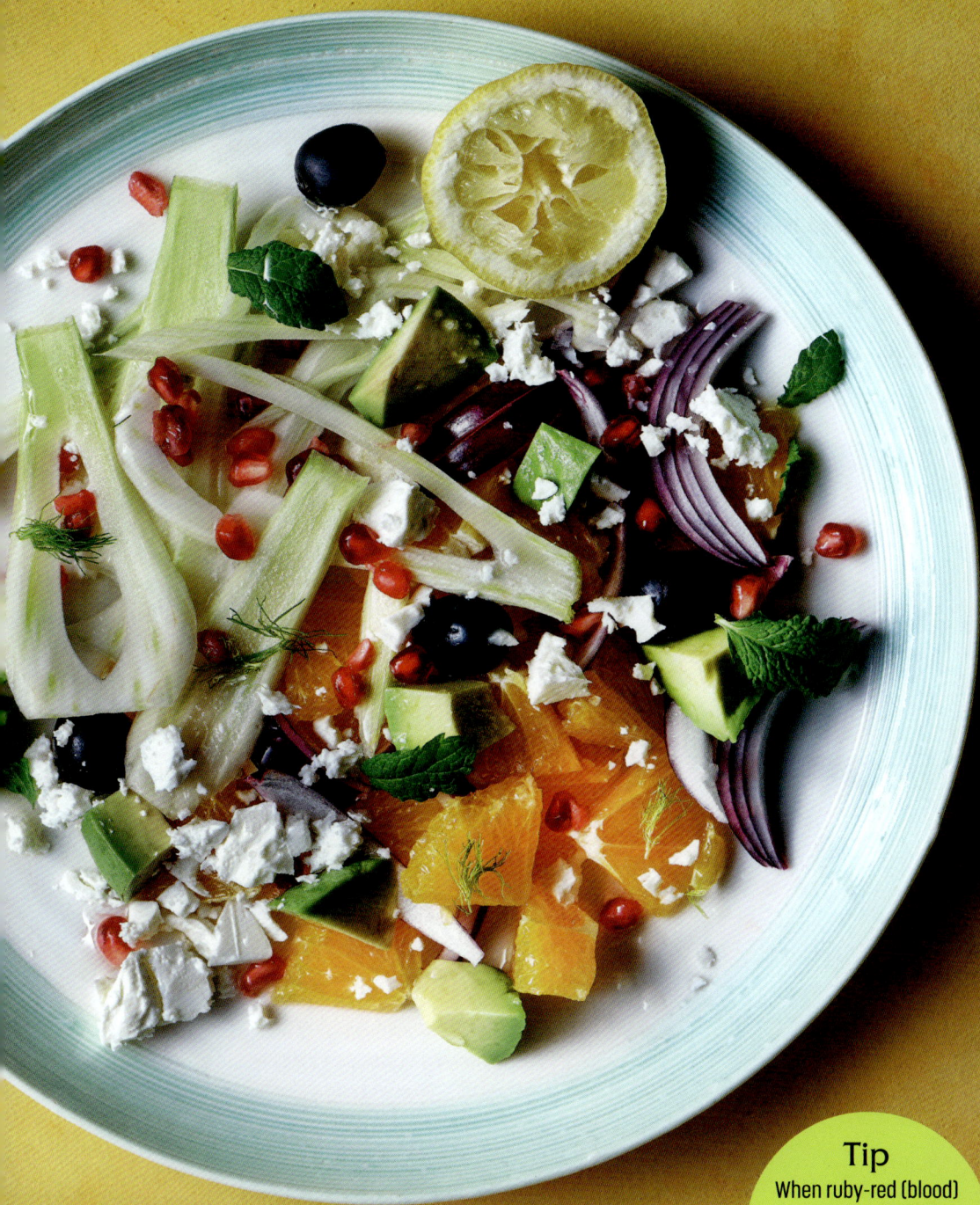

Tip
When ruby-red (blood) oranges are in season in late winter and early spring, they look spectacular in this salad.

HAWAIIAN-STYLE SALMON POKE BOWL

This tropical-inspired dish tastes as delicious as it looks. The perfectly balanced ingredients in this bowl of sunshine combine slow-releasing carbs with a host of antioxidants, which help zap free radicals (those rogue molecules that can damage your cells and cause ageing). The heart-healthy salmon is a treasure trove of omega-3 fats, which help to fight inflammation, protect your gut and support overall health.

SERVES
2

PREP
15
minutes

COOK
10–15
minutes

425
kcals
PER SERVING

60g brown rice (dry weight)
1 tbsp light soy sauce
1 tsp rice vinegar
½ tsp sesame oil
½ tsp caster sugar
180g good–quality skinless, boneless salmon fillet, cut into 2cm cubes
2 spring onions, finely sliced
shredded nori and sesame seeds, for sprinkling

For the salad
150g frozen shelled edamame beans
¼ cucumber, cubed
4 radishes, finely sliced
1 small avocado, peeled, stoned and cubed
large handful of baby spinach leaves
1 tbsp light soy sauce
1 tbsp rice vinegar
juice of ½ lime
1 tsp grated fresh root ginger

1. Cook the rice according to the instructions on the packet.

2. Meanwhile, whisk together the soy sauce, rice vinegar, sesame oil and sugar in a bowl until well combined. Gently stir in the salmon cubes and spring onions until everything is lightly coated.

3. To make the salad, cook the edamame beans in a pan of boiling water for 1 minute. Refresh under cold running water and drain well. Transfer to a salad bowl, along with the cucumber, radishes, avocado and spinach. In a small bowl or jug, whisk together the soy sauce, vinegar, lime juice and ginger, then pour this over the edamame mixture and toss lightly.

4. Fluff up the grains of rice with a fork and divide between two bowls. Add the marinated salmon and the edamame salad, and serve sprinkled with nori and sesame seeds.

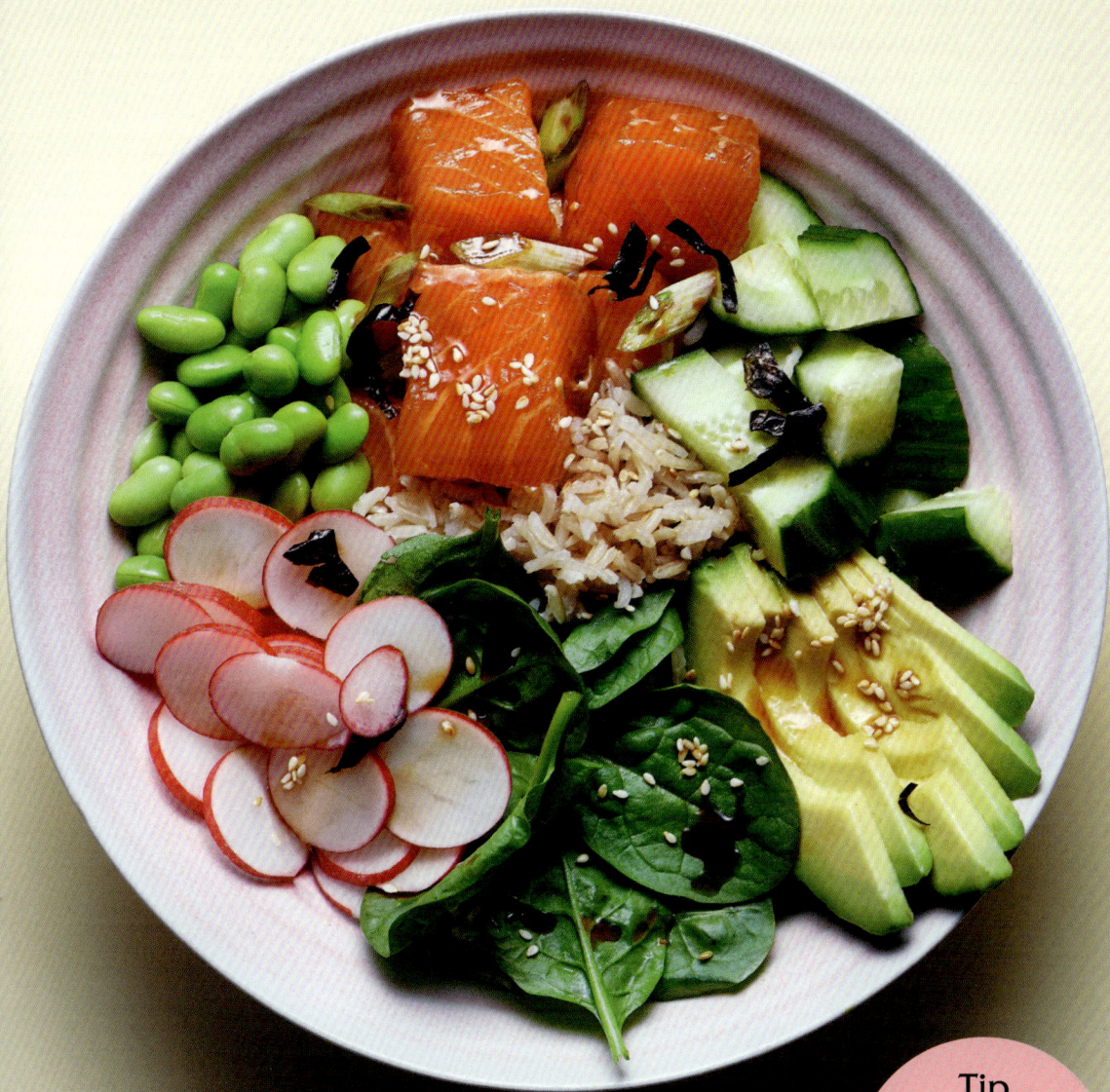

Tip
You can use good-quality raw tuna instead of salmon. If available, use sushi-quality fish.

NOTES
If you have time, you can soak the rice for at least 30 minutes before cooking. It's more time-consuming, but it makes it easier to digest.

NUTTY GRAIN BOWL

This nutty wholegrain bowl is packed with wholesome ingredients. Rich in fibre, vitamins and minerals, wholegrains offer numerous benefits for digestive health. We've included protein-rich tofu and a selection of vegetables, all topped with a delicious zesty dressing.

SERVES
2

PREP
10
minutes

COOK
9-10
minutes

435
kcals
PER SERVING

olive oil spray
80g long-stem broccoli, halved
1 yellow pepper, chopped
80g kale or spinach leaves, coarsely shredded
4 spring onions, sliced
100g firm or extra-firm tofu, cubed
2 tsp light soy sauce
100g cooked wholegrains from a pouch, such as spelt, quinoa or bulghur wheat
20g cashew nuts

200g canned chickpeas, rinsed and drained
a few flat-leaf parsley and/or mint sprigs, chopped
50g pomegranate seeds
sea salt and freshly ground black pepper

For the dressing
2 tsp olive oil
1 tsp balsamic or cider vinegar
juice of 1 lemon
1 tsp runny honey

1. Lightly spray a wok or frying pan with oil and set over a medium–high heat. Stir-fry the broccoli and yellow pepper for 2 minutes, then add the greens and spring onions and stir-fry for 1 minute more.

2. Toss the tofu in the soy sauce and add to the pan. Stir-fry for 4 minutes, until golden brown.

3. Add the wholegrains, cashews and chickpeas to the pan, and stir-fry for 1–2 minutes until warm. Remove from the heat and stir in the chopped herbs. Season to taste with salt and pepper.

4. To make the dressing, combine all the ingredients in a small bowl or jug, then pour over the grains and vegetables and toss to coat.

5. Divide between two serving bowls and sprinkle with pomegranate seeds. Eat hot or cold.

Tip
To make this bowl more substantial, crumble 60g feta cheese over the top.

NOTE
You can make this in advance, as it keeps well in an airtight container in the fridge for 24 hours.

CREAMY PASTA, HAM & SWEETCORN SALAD

You can't beat a quick, easy and delicious recipe for lunch. You'll probably have all these ingredients at home, which makes it a cinch to rustle up, and you can even make it in advance and pop it into the fridge for later. Our pasta salad has a light, tangy yogurt dressing, which adds healthy probiotics and a creamy flavour. The sweet cherry tomatoes and roasted peppers bring a burst of extra goodness.

SERVES
2

PREP
15
minutes

COOK
10–12
minutes

340
kcals
PER SERVING

60g farfalle or fusilli pasta (dry weight) (see tip)
60g frozen peas
100g lean boiled ham, diced
100g canned sweetcorn in water, drained
6 cherry tomatoes, halved
2 roasted red peppers from a jar, drained and sliced
2 spring onions, finely sliced

handful of flat-leaf parsley, chopped

For the yogurt Dijonnaise dressing
2 tbsp extra-light mayonnaise
3 tbsp fat-free Greek yogurt
1 tsp Dijon mustard
squeeze of lemon juice
sea salt and freshly ground black pepper

1. Cook the pasta in a large pan of boiling salted water according to the instructions on the packet. Drain and refresh in cold water, then drain in a colander.

2. Meanwhile, cook the frozen peas in a pan of boiling water for 2 minutes. Drain in a colander and set aside to cool.

3. To make the dressing, mix together all the ingredients in a bowl until well blended, and season to taste.

4. Put the pasta and peas into a large bowl and stir in the ham, sweetcorn, tomatoes, peppers and spring onions. Add the dressing and toss gently until everything is lightly coated, then sprinkle with parsley and serve.

Tip
You can use any dried pasta shapes you like, including penne or conchiglie. It's important that the pasta is perfectly cooked and holds its shape. For maximum fibre and nutritional goodness, use wholewheat (*integrale*) pasta.

LUNCHES

SWEET POTATO & CHICKPEA BUDDHA BOWL

This Buddha bowl is a treasure trove of health, bursting with the rich flavours of plant-based ingredients and packed full of nutritional benefits. Not only is it satisfying and fibre-rich, but it's also soothing for the soul! Sweet potatoes inject a dose of vitamins A and C, enhancing eye health and immunity, while chickpeas contribute protein and heart-healthy fibre, supporting muscle health and digestive wellness. No kale? No problem. Add some baby spinach or wild rocket with the roasted veggies just before serving for a nutrient-packed twist.

SERVES
2

PREP
5
minutes

COOK
30
minutes

390
kcals
PER SERVING

1 small red onion, cut into wedges
200g sweet potato, peeled and cubed
100g cherry tomatoes
2 whole garlic cloves, unpeeled
a few thyme and rosemary sprigs
olive oil spray
100g kale, trimmed and any large stems removed

2 tbsp freshly chopped flat-leaf parsley
80g quinoa (dry weight)
100g Spicy Air-fried Chickpeas (see page 104)
4 tbsp fat-free Greek yogurt
2 tsp sweet chilli sauce (optional)
sea salt and freshly ground black pepper

1. Preheat the oven to 200°C (gas mark 6).

2. Combine the onion, sweet potato and tomatoes in a large roasting tray. Tuck in the garlic cloves and herb sprigs, and spray with olive oil. Season with salt and pepper and roast for 25 minutes, or until the vegetables are tender. Stir the kale into the roasted vegetables and roast for a further 5 minutes. Remove the tray from the oven and discard the herbs. Squeeze the garlic cloves out of their skins and stir into the roasted vegetable mixture, along with the chopped parsley.

3. Meanwhile, cook the quinoa according to the instructions on the packet.

4. Divide the spicy chickpeas, roasted vegetables and quinoa between two bowls. Top with the yogurt and drizzle with chilli sauce (if using), then serve.

Tip
It's so easy to air-fry or roast some spicy chickpeas, but if you don't have the time, you can substitute some drained canned ones instead.

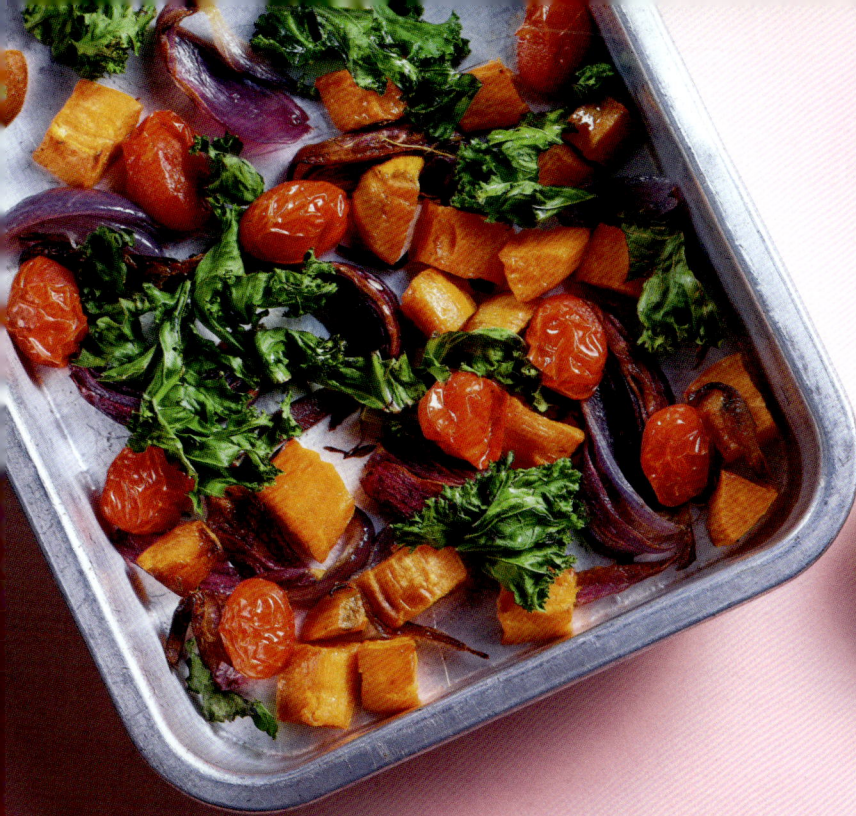

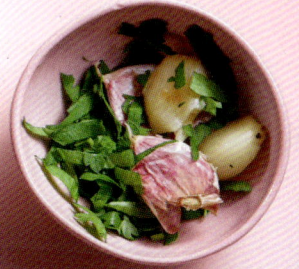

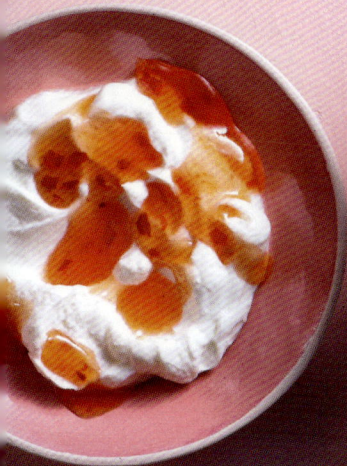

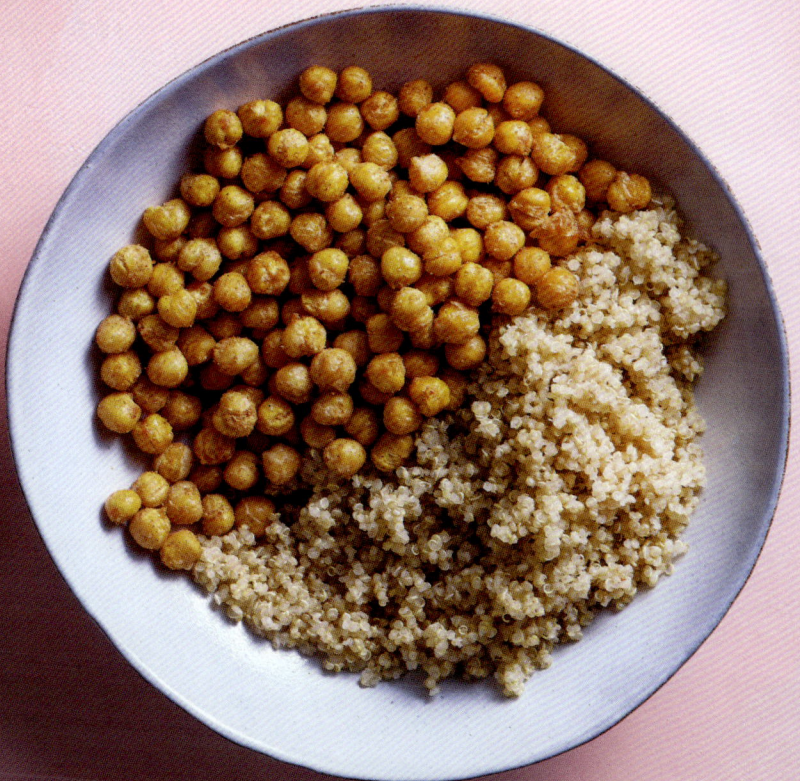

MYKONOS-STYLE ORZO SALAD

At first glance, orzo might look like grains of rice, but it's actually a type of pasta. It's often served as a salad in Greece, especially during the summer months, with colourful vegetables and feta or soft goat's cheese. Here we've created a delicious balance of orzo (for slow energy release) with vibrant vegetables and a drizzle of light pesto. It's sunshine on a plate, and a hug for your gut.

SERVES
2

PREP
10
minutes

COOK
8–10
minutes

345
kcals
PER SERVING

60g orzo (dry weight)
1 tsp fruity green olive oil
60g baby spinach leaves
6 cherry or baby plum
   tomatoes, quartered
2 spring onions, finely sliced
6 Kalamata olives, pitted
20g pine nuts

60g feta cheese, crumbled
a few fresh basil leaves, torn
sea salt and freshly ground
   black pepper

For the pesto dressing
juice of ½ small lemon
2 tsp red wine vinegar
2 tbsp green pesto

1. Cook the orzo according to the instructions on the packet. Drain well and transfer to a bowl. Toss in the olive oil, then set aside to cool until it's just lukewarm.

2. Meanwhile, make the pesto dressing by mixing together the ingredients in a jug or small bowl.

3. Pour the dressing over the orzo and gently toss until the pasta grains are lightly coated. Stir in the spinach, tomatoes, spring onions, olives and pine nuts. Season to taste (remember that feta is quite salty, so go easy on the salt), then crumble the feta over the top. Serve warm or at room temperature, sprinkled with basil.

NOTES
If you want to enjoy this as a packed lunch, transport the spinach leaves in a separate container and add to the salad just before eating.

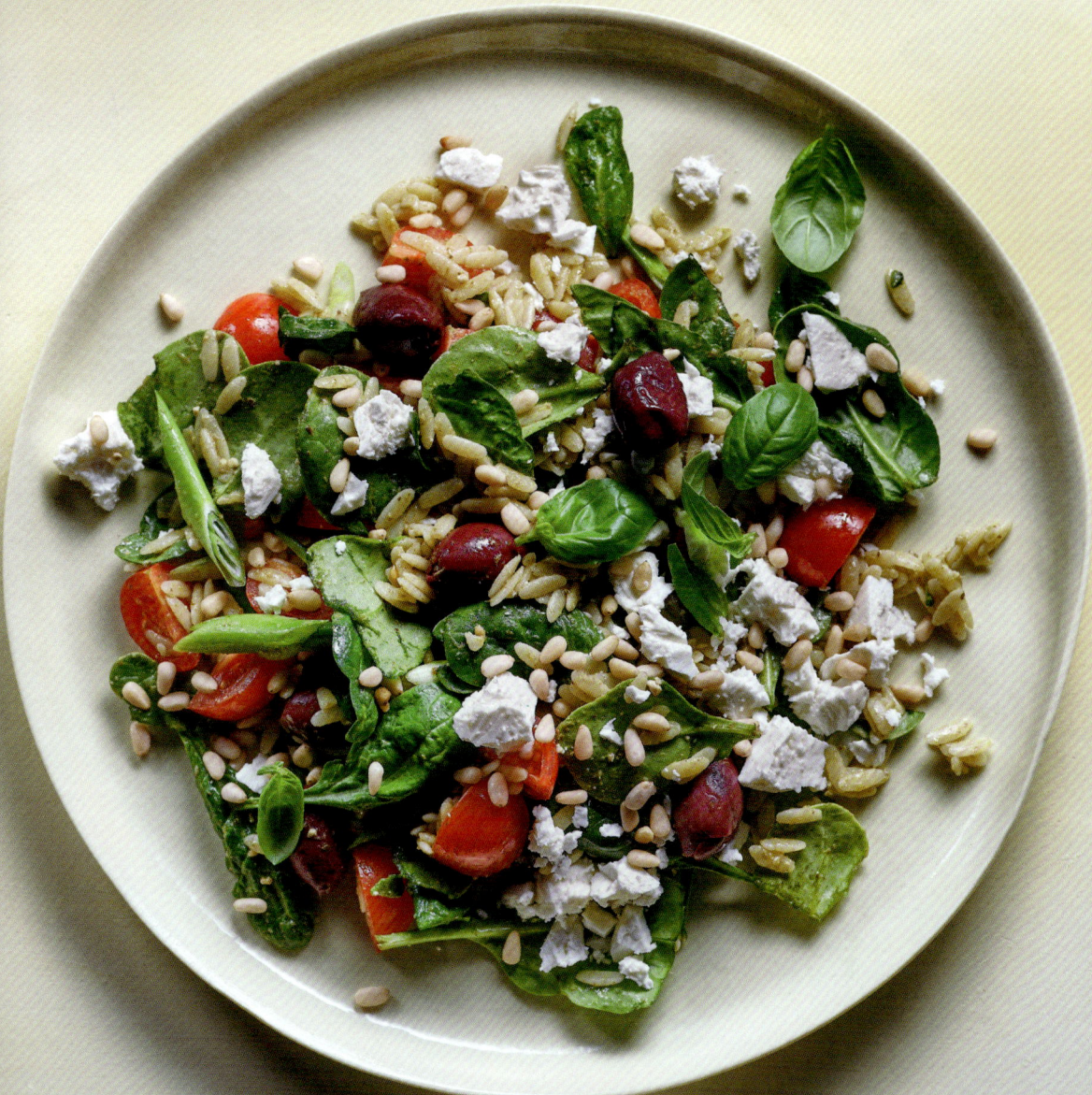

Tip

Orzo is usually made from wheat, but gluten-free alternatives are also available.

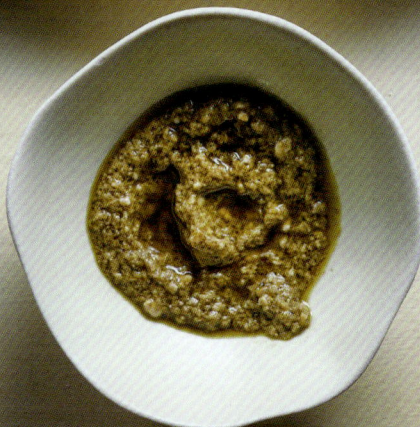

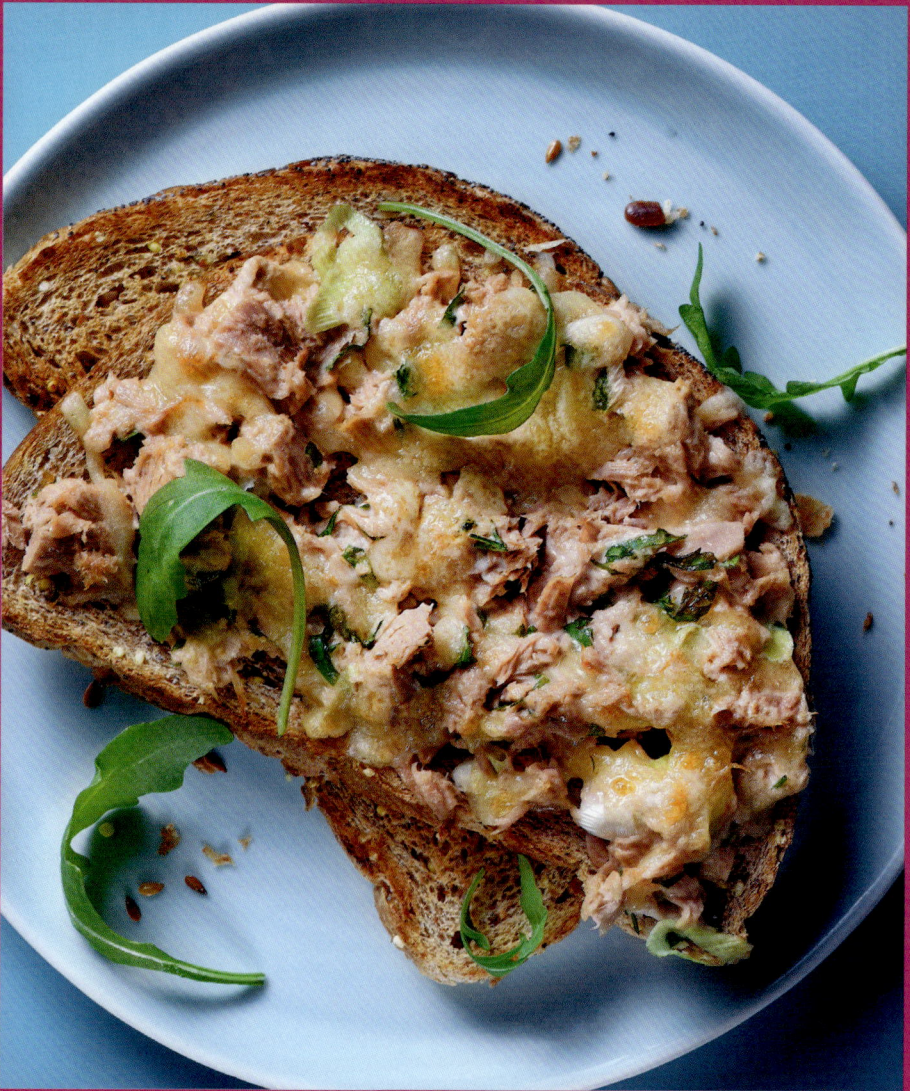

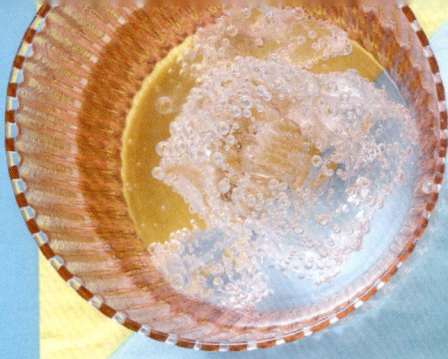

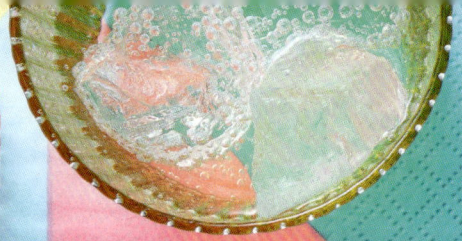

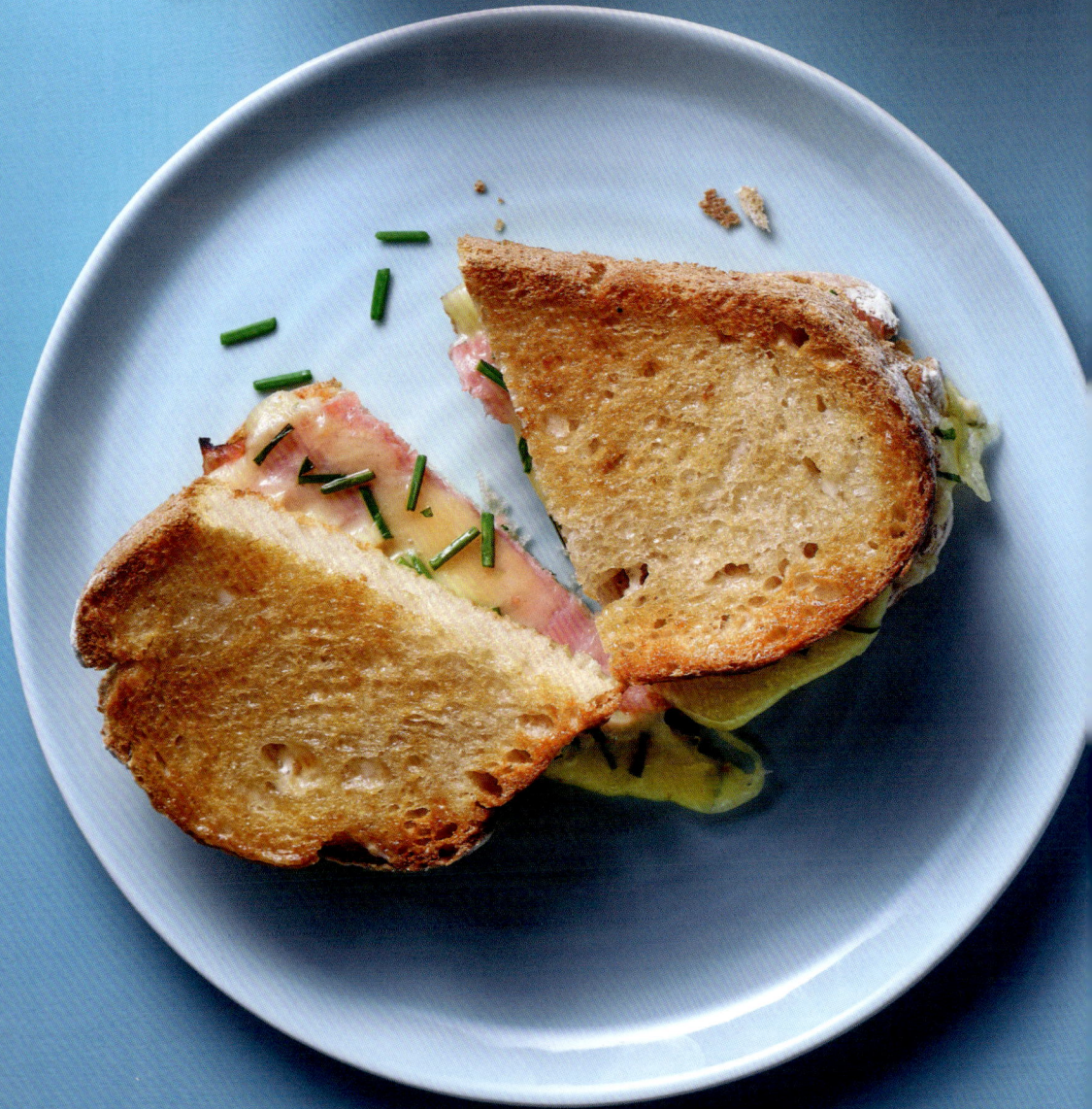

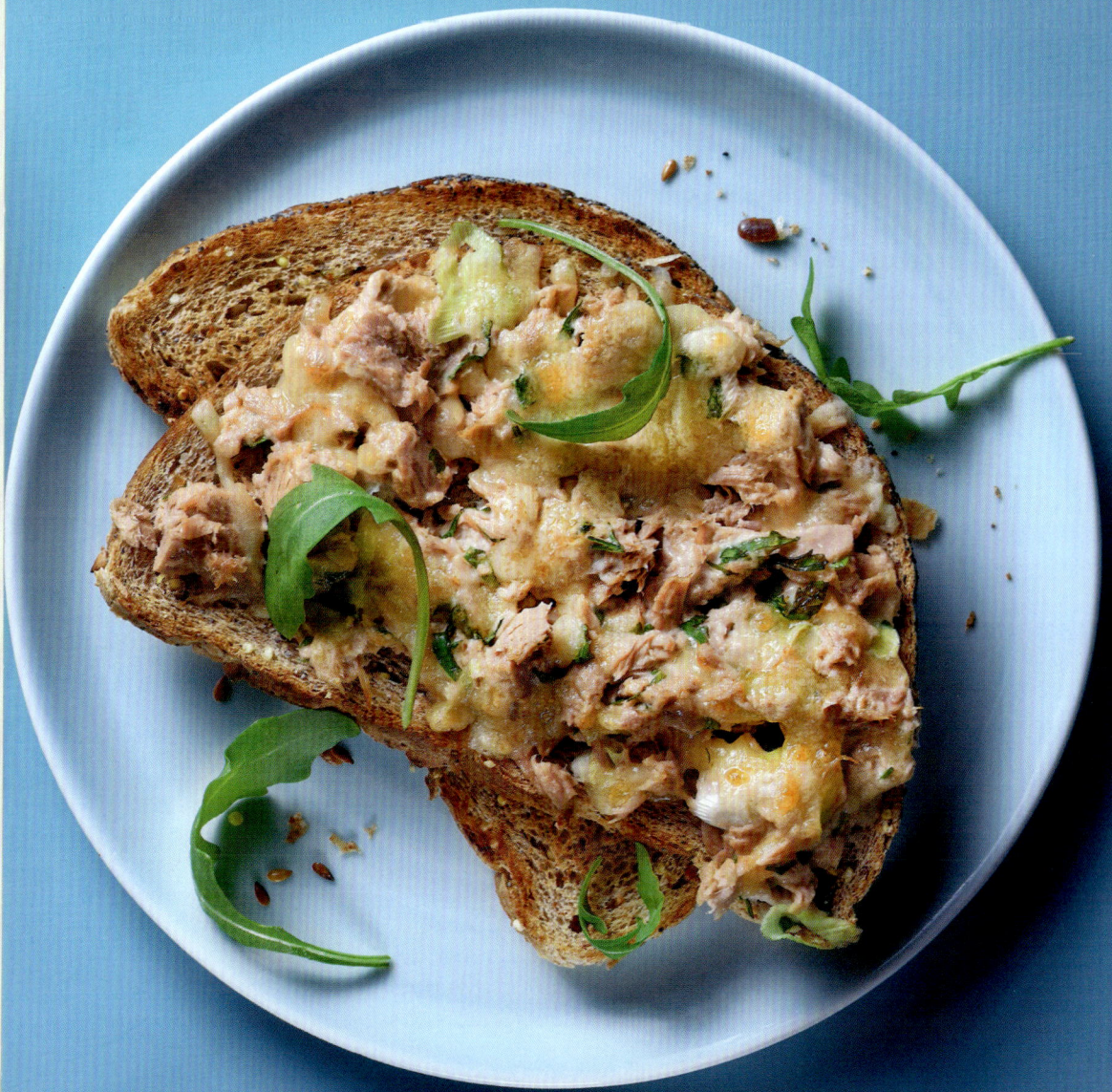

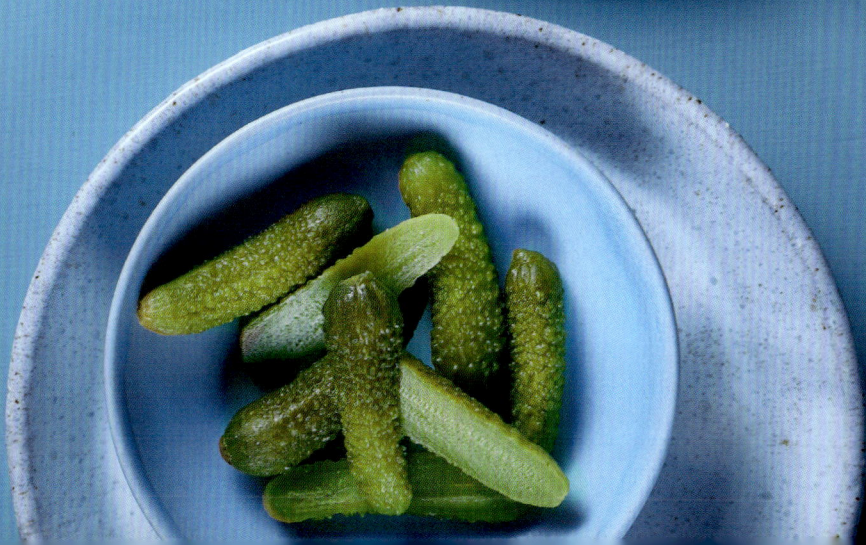

GRILLED TOFU GYROS with tzatziki (continued)

3. Lightly spray the aubergine slices with oil on both sides. Sprinkle with oregano and season with salt and pepper. Set a ridged non-stick griddle pan over a medium–high heat and cook the aubergine, in batches, for 2–3 minutes on each side, until golden brown and striped. Drain on a plate lined with kitchen paper and keep warm.

4. Remove the tofu from the marinade and drain on kitchen paper. Lightly spray the hot griddle pan with oil and add the tofu (if your pan isn't large, do this in batches). Cook over a medium–high heat for 3 minutes on each side until golden and crispy. Remove and drain on a plate lined with kitchen paper.

5. Heat the wraps in the griddle pan, then divide the aubergine, tofu, cucumber, tomatoes, onion and lettuce between them. Spoon the tzatziki over the top, adding a dash of harissa. Place each wrap on a square of foil or baking parchment and roll. Eat immediately.

Tip
Feel free to swap aubergine for 2 red or yellow peppers and cook in the griddle pan in the same way.

EASY BEANY BURRITOS

These burritos, filled with pulses, fresh salad and yogurt, can be enjoyed heated or chilled — they're a fantastic pick for a lunch box. Beans, along with other legumes, stand out as some of the most nutrient-rich plant foods available. Recent studies indicate that regular consumption of these foods is associated with better health and increased longevity. Avocados bring a rich, creamy texture to the mix, along with beneficial vitamins and minerals, enhancing your gut health with each bite.

SERVES
2

PREP
10
minutes

COOK
8
minutes

460
kcals
PER SERVING

olive oil spray
4 spring onions, sliced
1 red pepper, diced
200g canned black beans, drained and rinsed
½ tsp chilli powder
½ tsp paprika
2 wholewheat tortillas (about 40g each)
handful of crisp lettuce leaves, shredded
60g Cheddar cheese, grated
2 tbsp fat-free Greek yogurt

sea salt and freshly ground black pepper

For the avocado chilli smash
1 small ripe avocado, peeled and stoned
1 tomato, diced
1 red chilli, diced
½ tsp chilli powder
juice of ½ lime
handful of coriander, chopped
2 tbsp hot tomato salsa

1. Lightly spray a frying pan with oil and set over a low–medium heat. Add the spring onions and red pepper and cook, stirring occasionally, for 3 minutes or until softened. Stir in the beans, chilli powder and paprika, and heat through for 5 minutes. Season to taste.

2. Meanwhile, make the avocado chilli smash. Coarsely mash the avocado in a bowl and stir in the other ingredients. Season to taste.

3. Warm the tortillas in a lightly oiled griddle pan set over a low heat.

4. Spread the bean mixture over the warm tortillas and cover with the lettuce. Spoon on the smashed avocado, and top with the grated cheese and yogurt.

5. Roll up the tortillas or fold in the sides and ends to enclose the filling. Enjoy!

Tip
If you don't have black beans, use kidney beans or chickpeas instead. For a really authentic flavour, use Mexican red jalapeño chilli powder.

GRILLED CHICKEN TACOS

You can enjoy these tacos straight from the griddle or chilled, making them perfect for a grab-and-go lunch. The pickled red onion adds a sweet tanginess, and your gut will love the fermentation perks they bring. Sweetcorn adds a satisfying crunch to each bite. You can use homemade or shop-bought guacamole – it's all good. And if you're out of guac, simply mashing up half a small avocado will do the trick beautifully.

SERVES
2

PREP
15
minutes

COOK
12–15
minutes

405
kcals
PER SERVING

olive oil spray
200g skinless chicken breast fillets
1 tsp Mexican-style or taco seasoning
juice of 1 lime
handful of coriander, chopped
60g canned sweetcorn in water, drained
2 tomatoes, chopped
1 red chilli, diced
2 wholemeal wraps (about 40g each)

handful of crisp lettuce leaves, shredded
2 heaped tbsp guacamole
sea salt and freshly ground black pepper

For the pickled red onion
50ml red wine vinegar
20g caster sugar
large pinch of salt
1 small red onion, finely sliced

1. To make the pickled red onion, combine all the ingredients except the onion in a small pan set over a low–medium heat. Add 2 tbsp water and stir well until the sugar dissolved. Bring to the boil and let it bubble for 1 minute, then take it off the heat. Stir in the onion and set aside until cool.

2. Lightly spray a frying pan with oil and set over a medium–high heat. Toss the chicken in the Mexican-style or taco seasoning, then add to the pan. Cook for 12–15 minutes, turning once or twice, until seared and golden and cooked right through.

3. Cut the chicken into chunks and transfer to a bowl. Sprinkle with the lime juice and coriander, and season with salt and pepper. Stir in the sweetcorn, tomatoes and chilli.

4. Warm the wraps in a lightly oiled griddle pan or low oven. Cover with the lettuce and the chicken mixture, followed by the guacamole. Top with a spoonful of pickled red onions and roll or fold to enclose the filling. Enjoy.

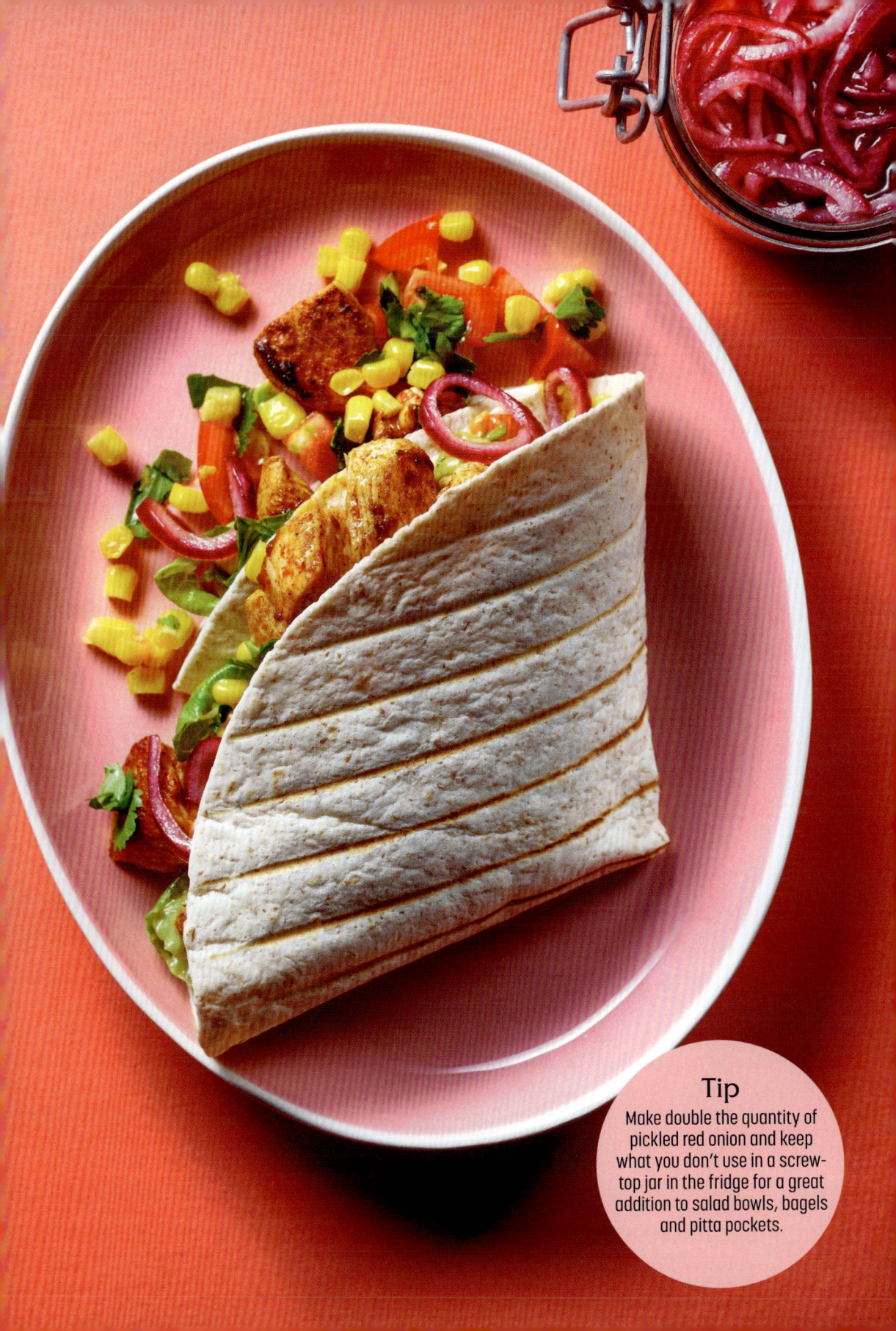

Tip
Make double the quantity of pickled red onion and keep what you don't use in a screw-top jar in the fridge for a great addition to salad bowls, bagels and pitta pockets.

CHICKEN WRAPS
with green goddess dressing

These wraps are heavenly: spiced chicken and griddled peppers rolled up with the best green salad you'll ever taste. They are best served warm, but are still delicious if you make them in advance and enjoy them cold as a packed lunch. Packed with protein, vitamins, minerals and dietary fibre, they will make your gut very happy.

SERVES
2

PREP
15
minutes

COOK
10–12
minutes

400
kcals
PER SERVING

Tip
Stir some snipped chives into the green goddess dressing after blitzing.

olive oil spray
200g skinless chicken breast fillets, cut into strips
1 red pepper, cut into strips
2 garlic cloves, crushed
1 red chilli, deseeded and finely sliced
handful of crisp lettuce leaves
2 spring onions, sliced
¼ cucumber, diced
1 small ripe avocado, peeled, stoned and cubed

2 wholemeal wraps (about 40g each)
sea salt and freshly ground black pepper

For the green goddess dressing
2 tbsp light mayonnaise
2 tbsp fat-free Greek yogurt
handful of flat-leaf parsley
handful of basil leaves
1 tsp lemon juice
1 anchovy fillet, drained

1. To make the green goddess dressing, blitz everything in a blender until smooth and green. Season with salt and pepper to taste. Add more lemon juice if wished.

2. Lightly spray a frying pan with oil and set over a medium heat. Add the chicken and red pepper and cook, turning occasionally, for 10 minutes, or until the chicken is golden brown and cooked right through, and the pepper is tender. Stir in the garlic and chilli and cook for 1 minute more.

3. Meanwhile, in a bowl, mix the lettuce, spring onions, cucumber and avocado. Pour over the dressing and toss until everything is lightly coated.

4. Heat the wraps in the microwave or warm them in a griddle pan set over a low to medium heat.

5. Divide the chicken and peppers between the wraps and top with the green goddess dressing. Fold or roll the wraps to enclose the filling, then serve.

CRUNCHY CARROT & FALAFEL WRAPS

Ideal for a workday lunch, our vibrant, wholesome wraps are satisfying and nutritious, and can be rustled up easily in less than 20 minutes. The wholemeal wraps, creamy hummus, zesty falafel seeds and crunchy fresh veggies bring a gut-loving fibre-feast to your body and will power you up all afternoon.

SERVES
2

PREP
10
minutes

COOK
8
minutes

450
kcals
PER SERVING

olive oil spray
1 small red onion, finely sliced
2 large carrots, peeled and cut into matchsticks
2 garlic cloves, crushed
1 red bird's-eye chilli, shredded
1 tsp caraway seeds
1 tsp cumin seeds
2 × wholemeal wraps (about 40g each)

100g hummus
6 falafels (see tip)
4 tbsp fat-free Greek yogurt (or dairy-free yogurt)
a few flat-leaf parsley sprigs, chopped
2 tsp sweet chilli sauce
sea salt and freshly ground black pepper

1. Lightly spray a frying pan with oil and set over a medium heat. Add the onion, carrots, garlic and chilli, along with the caraway and cumin seeds. Cook, stirring occasionally, for 8 minutes, or until the onion softens and the carrot is tender but still slightly crunchy. Season with salt and pepper.

2. Meanwhile, warm the wraps on a hot griddle pan or in a low oven.

3. Spread the hummus over the wraps and pile the carrot mixture on top, followed by the falafels. Add the yogurt and sprinkle with parsley. Drizzle with sweet chilli sauce, roll up and enjoy.

Tip
You don't have to make your own falafel; most supermarkets and delis sell them. Just check the labels before buying and avoid any that include ultra processed ingredients.

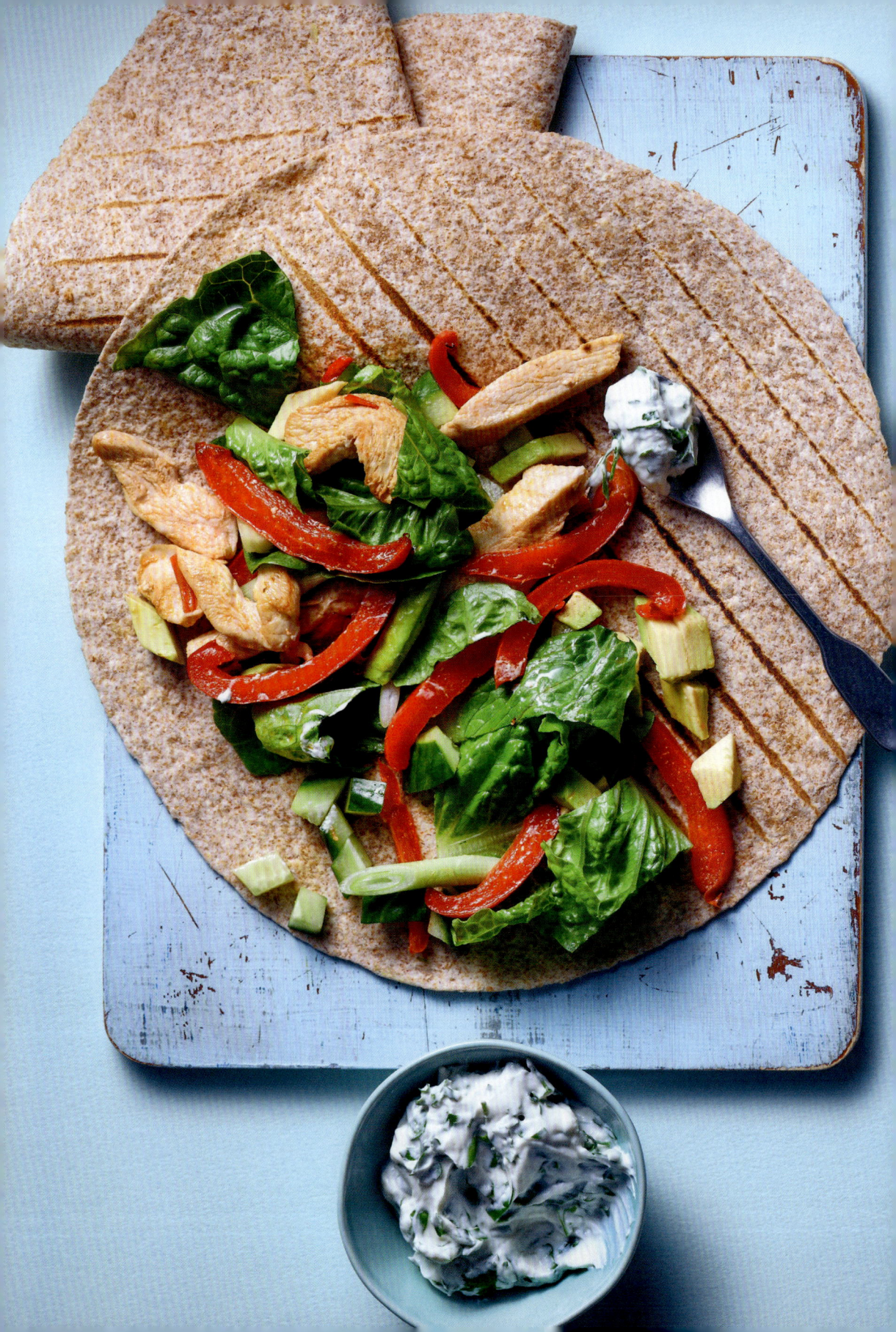

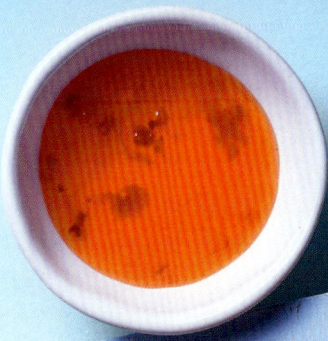

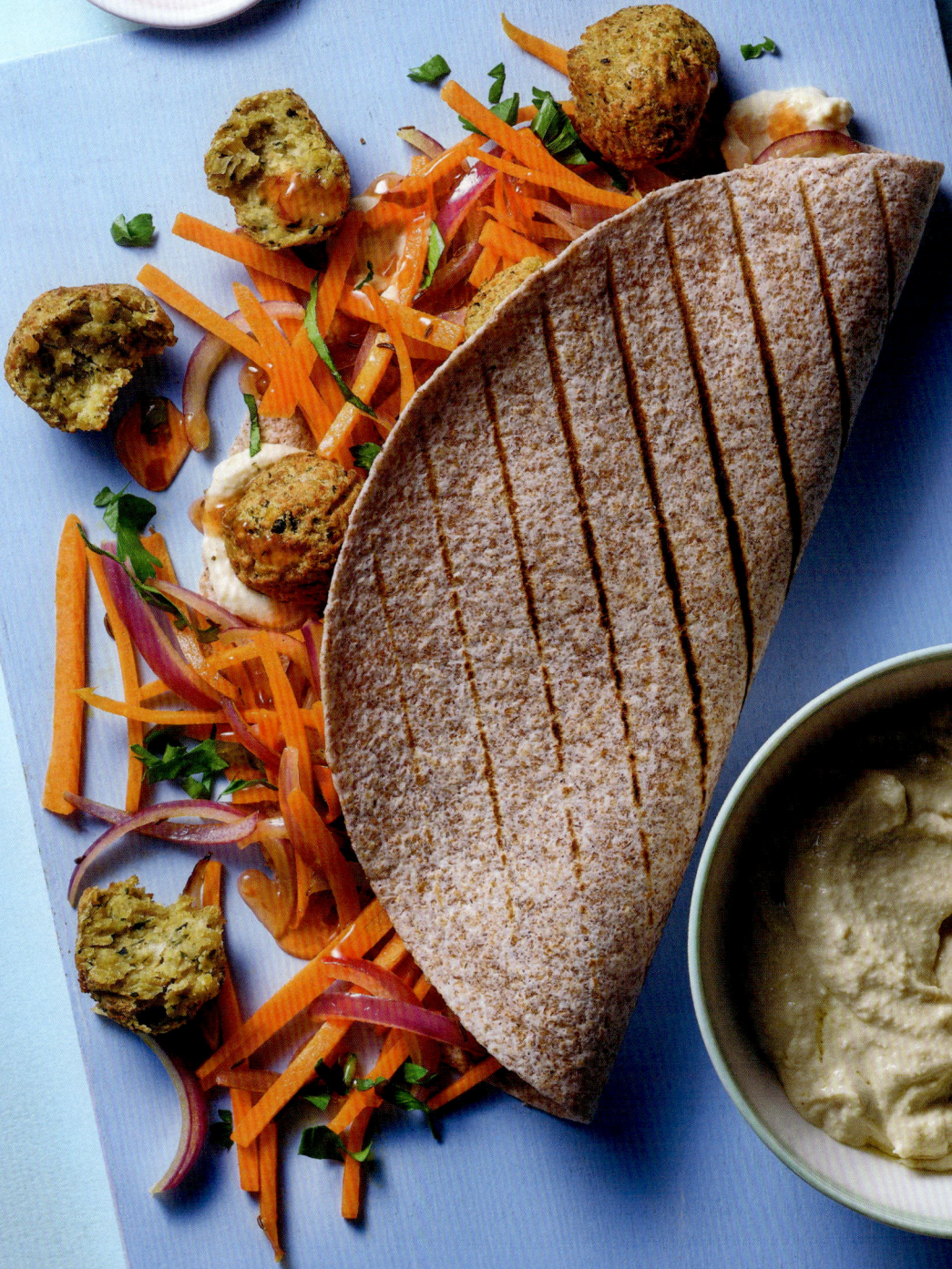

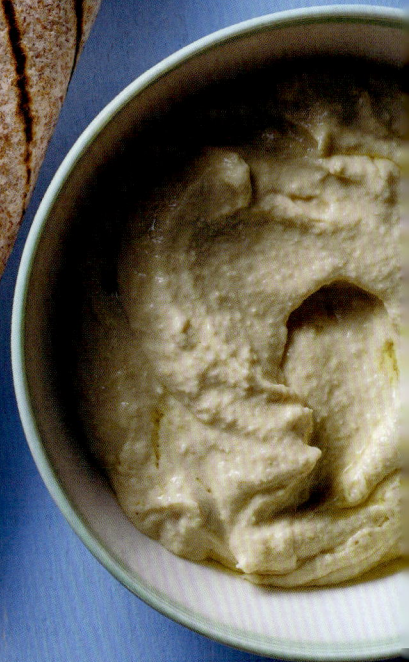

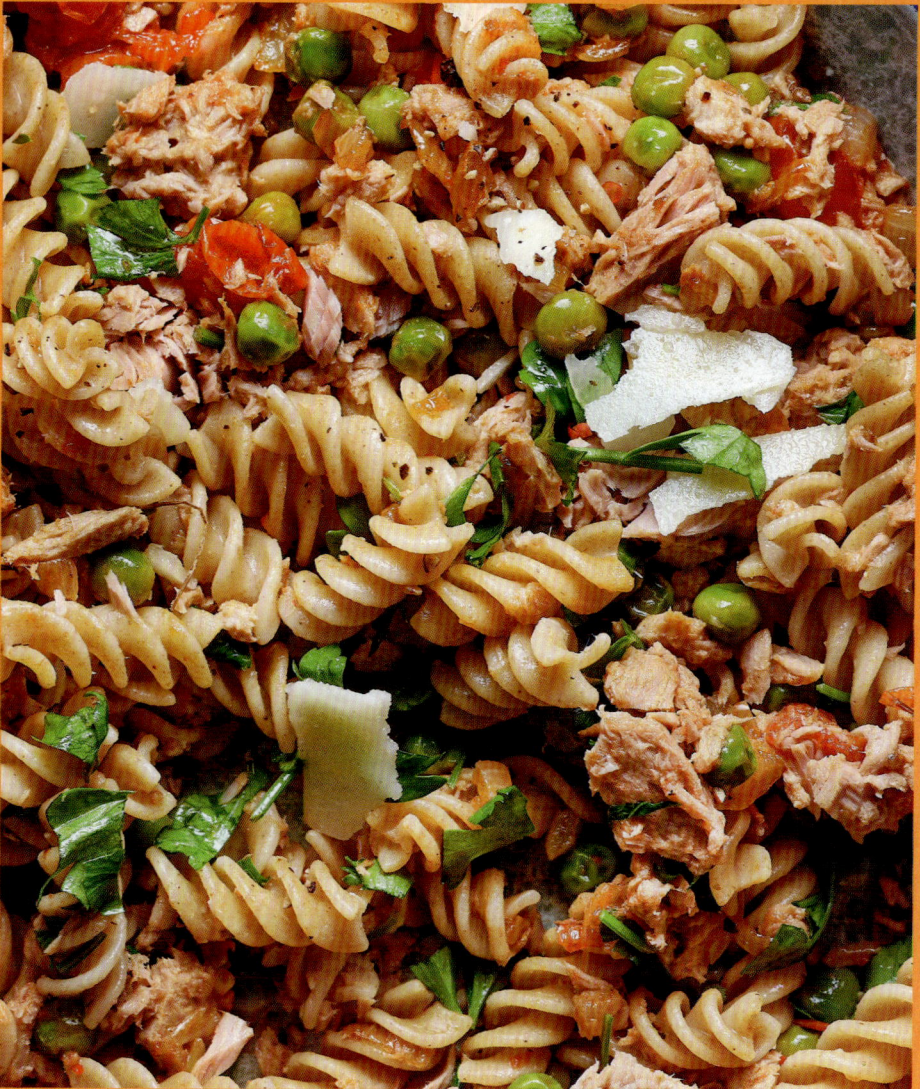

AUBERGINE PIZZA SLICES

A super-healthy way to make mini pizzas is to use griddled vegetables for the base – smoky-tasting aubergines work particularly well. They're low in calories, antioxidant-rich and are adored by your microbiome! Feel free to be creative with the toppings based on what veggies you have in your fridge.

SERVES
2

PREP
10
minutes

COOK
15–20
minutes

300
kcals
PER SERVING

2 large aubergines, ends trimmed
olive oil spray
2 juicy tomatoes, finely sliced
pinch of dried oregano
a few baby spinach leaves
100g mozzarella, grated or sliced
¼ red onion, finely sliced
1 red or yellow pepper, finely sliced
1 tbsp green pesto
sea salt and freshly ground black pepper
crisp green salad, to serve

1. Preheat the oven to 200°C (gas mark 6).

2. Cut each aubergine lengthways into 3 thick slices and lightly spray them with oil on both sides. Season with salt and pepper.

3. Place a ridged non-stick griddle pan over a medium–high heat, and when it's hot, add some of the aubergine slices. Cook for 2–3 minutes until golden brown and attractively striped underneath, then turn them over and cook on the other side. Set aside on a plate lined with kitchen paper to drain and keep warm while you griddle the rest.

4. Place the griddled aubergine slices on a baking tray and arrange the sliced tomatoes over them. Sprinkle with the oregano and spinach leaves. Cover with the mozzarella and top with the finely sliced onion and red or yellow pepper. Season with salt and pepper and spray lightly with oil.

5. Bake for 6–8 minutes, or until the cheese is bubbling and golden brown and the vegetables are tender.

6. Using a fish slice, carefully remove the aubergine pizza slices to two serving plates. Drizzle with pesto and serve piping hot with a crisp green salad.

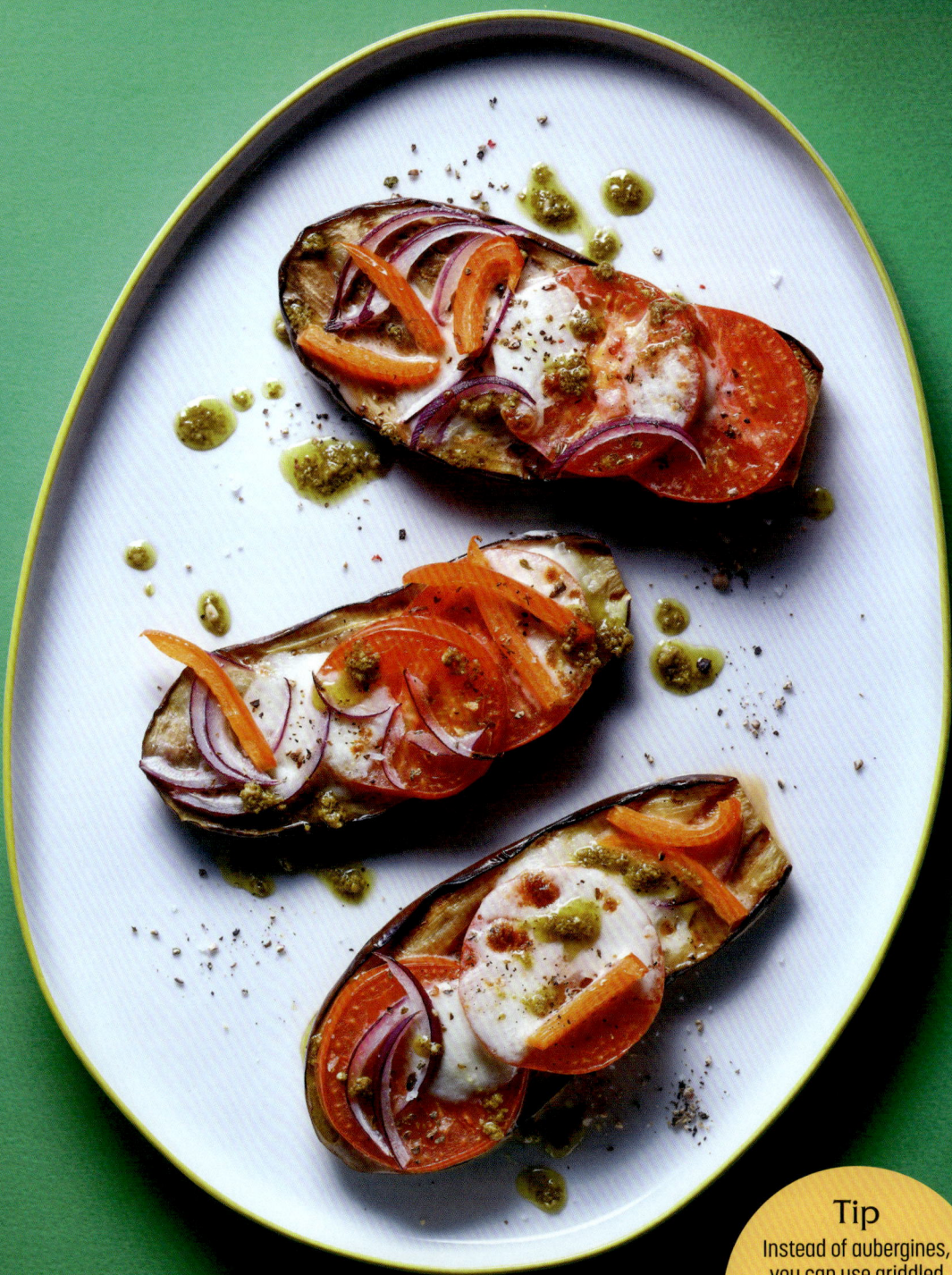

Tip
Instead of aubergines, you can use griddled sweet potato, courgettes or even Portobello mushrooms for the pizza 'bases'.

EASY-PEASY TUNA PASTA

Pressed for time? This speedy lunch has got you covered! With just a quick chop of an onion, you're 15 minutes away from a delicious pasta meal. Onions and garlic bring a rich, savoury depth to pasta creations, plus they're gut-health champions thanks to their remarkable health-boosting properties. Paired with canned tuna's lean protein, vital for the repair and growth of body tissues and a healthy digestive system, you've got a speedy, nutritious meal that's hard to beat. Chances are, you already have everything you need in your pantry, fridge and freezer.

SERVES
2

PREP
5
minutes

COOK
15
minutes

290
kcals
PER SERVING

olive oil spray
1 onion, diced
3 garlic cloves, crushed
8 baby plum or cherry
tomatoes
1 tsp tomato purée
160g can tuna in natural spring
water, drained and roughly
flaked
60g frozen peas

60g wholewheat pasta, such as
penne or fusilli (dry weight)
squeeze of lemon juice
(optional)
a few flat-leaf parsley sprigs,
chopped
4 tbsp grated Parmesan cheese
sea salt and freshly ground
black pepper

1. Lightly spray a frying pan with oil and set over a medium heat. Add the onion and garlic and cook, stirring occasionally, for 5 minutes, or until tender but not browned.

2. Add the tomatoes and cook for 5 minutes more. As they start to soften, press down on them with a spatula to squash them and release their juice. Stir in the tomato purée, and then add the tuna and frozen peas. Cook gently for 5 minutes until the peas are tender. Season with salt and pepper to taste.

3. Meanwhile, cook the pasta in a pan of salted boiling water according to the instructions on the packet. Drain well.

4. Stir the pasta into the tuna and tomato mixture, add a squeeze of lemon juice (if wished) and sprinkle with parsley. Divide between two shallow bowls and serve immediately, topped with the Parmesan.

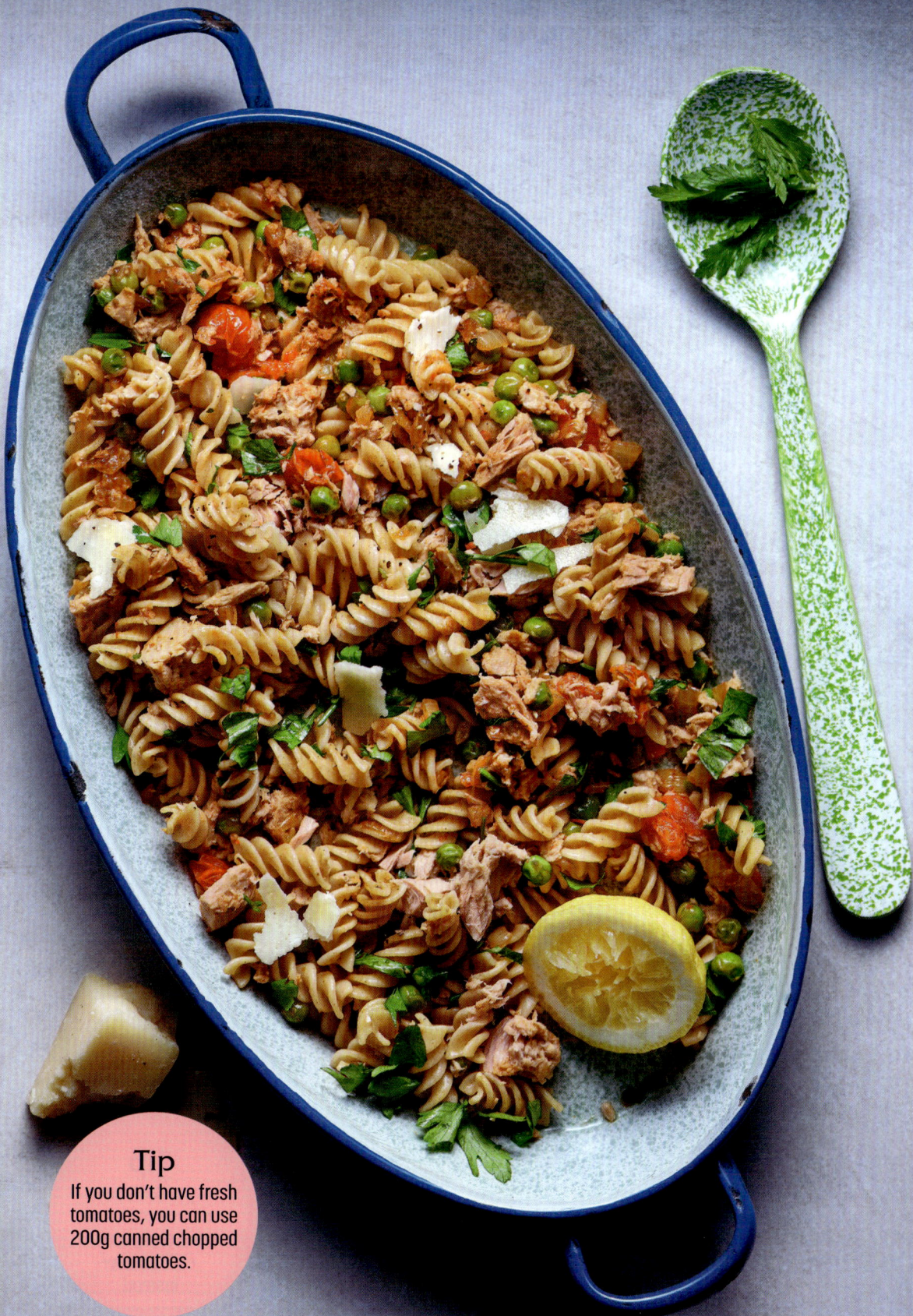

Tip
If you don't have fresh tomatoes, you can use 200g canned chopped tomatoes.

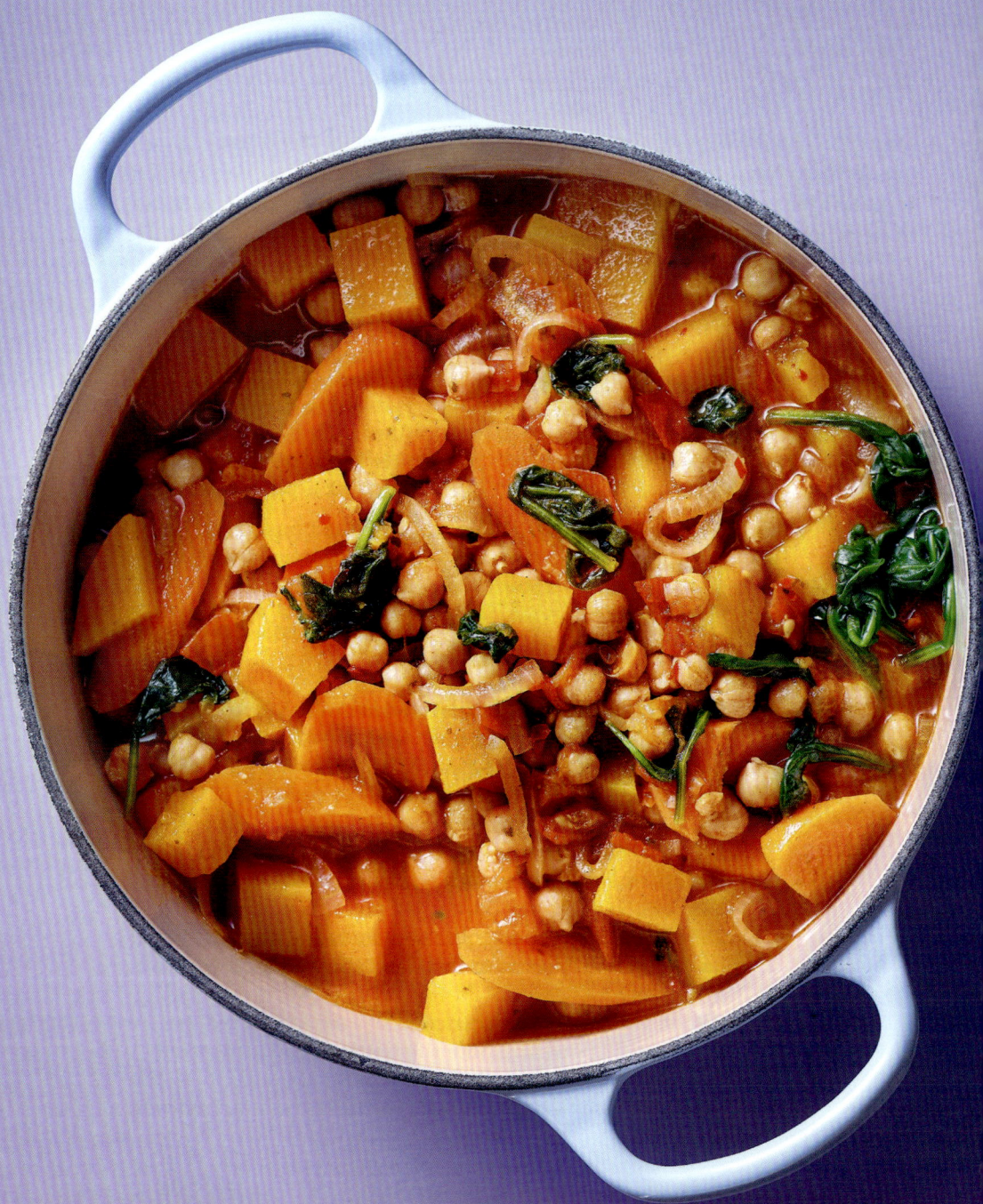

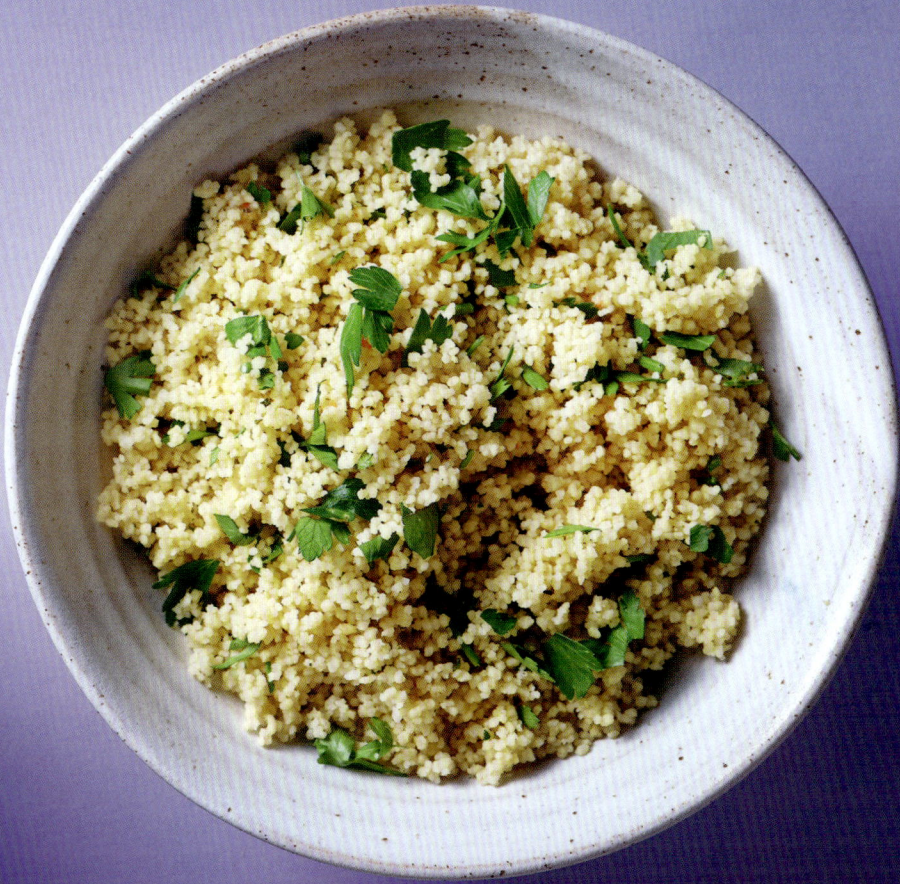

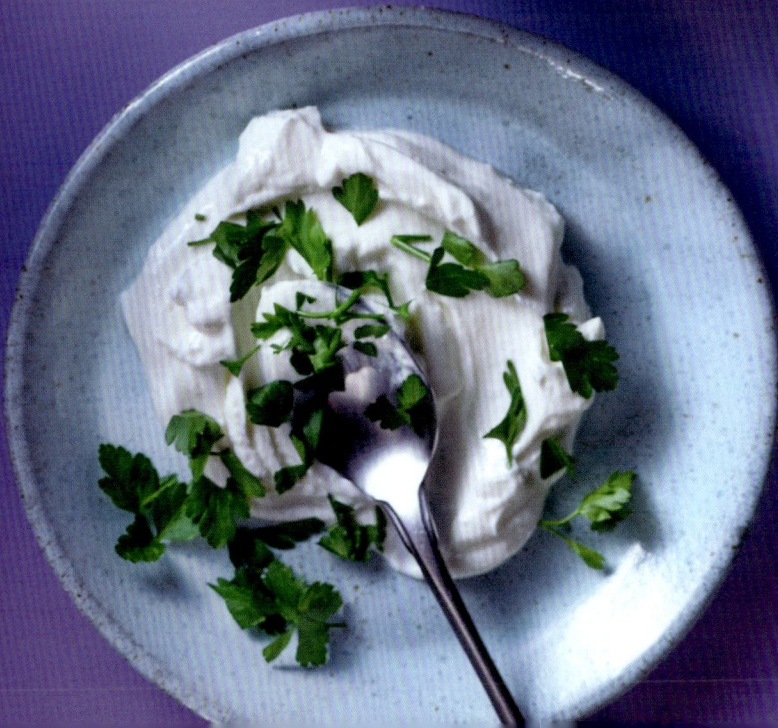

snacks

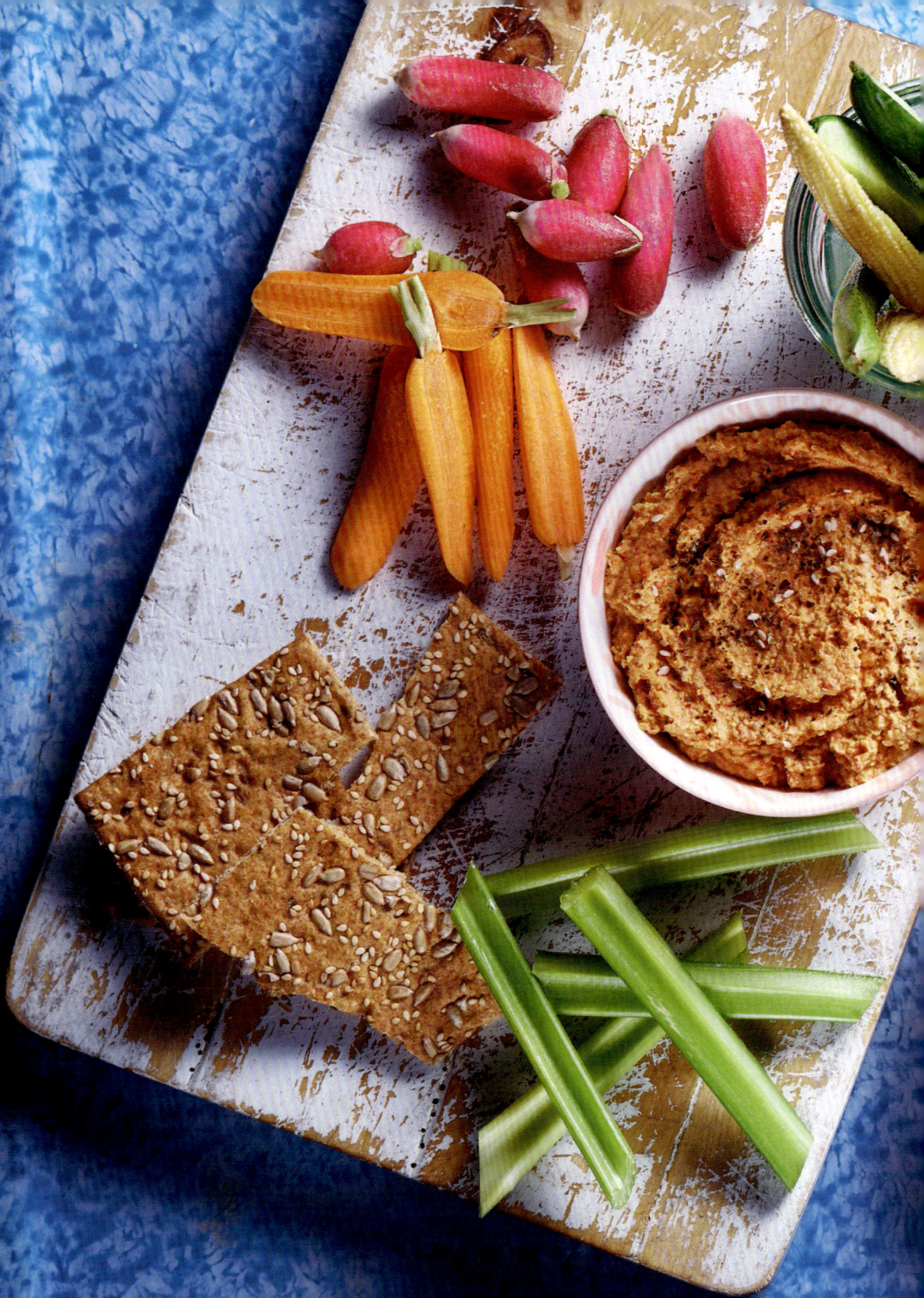

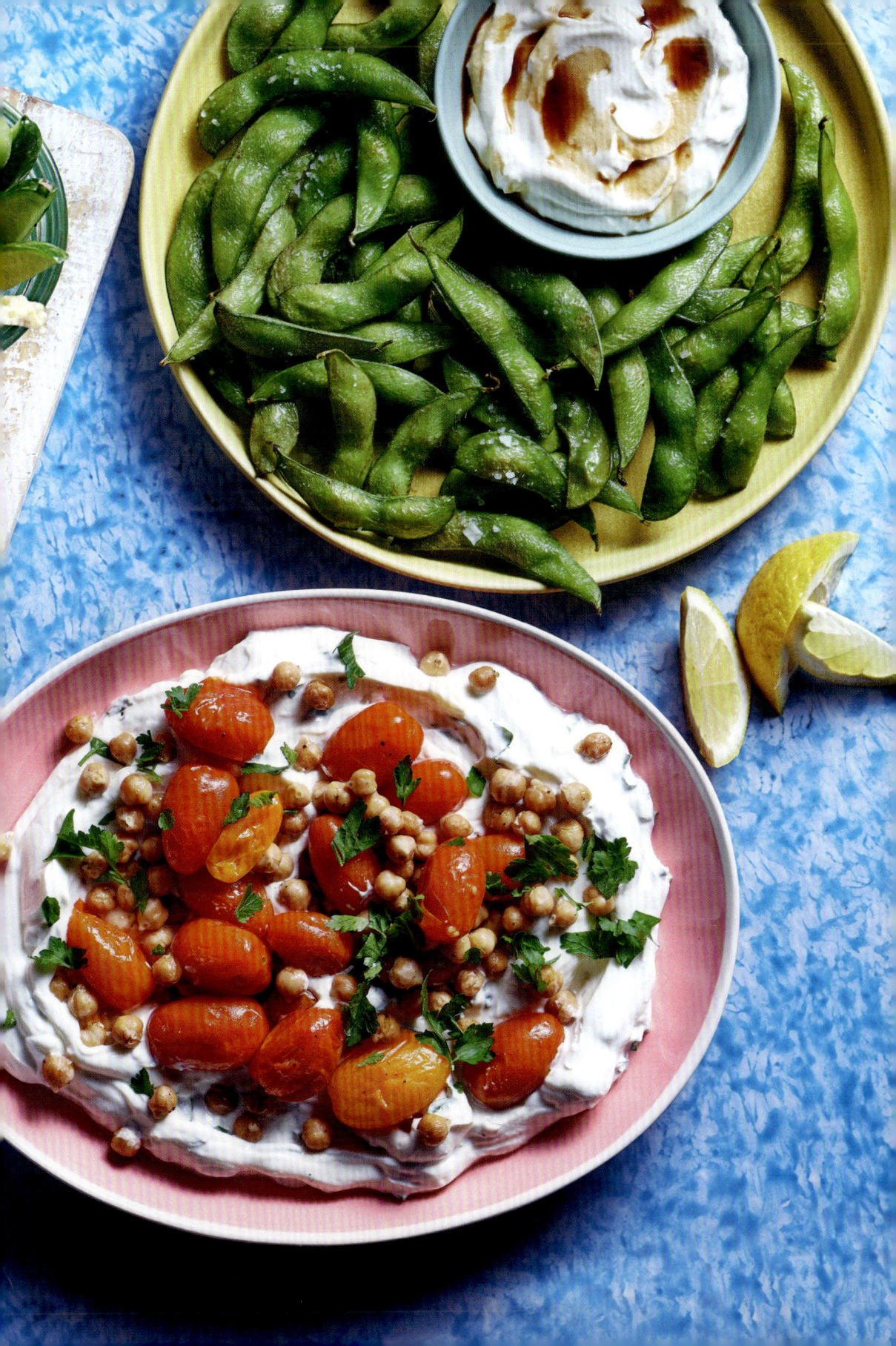

SPEEDY SOURDOUGH BRUSCHETTA

Bruschetta is always a good idea for a tasty snack. If you don't have sourdough, use wholegrain or wholemeal bread instead. Have fun experimenting with different gut-friendly toppings – to start you off, see Alternative Toppings below.

SERVES
2

PREP
10
minutes

COOK
2–3
minutes

220
kcals
PER SERVING

1 small ripe avocado, peeled and stoned
2 tbsp fat-free Greek yogurt
squeeze of lime juice
2 slices of sourdough (about 30g each), halved
olive oil spray
50g finely sliced smoked salmon

sea salt and freshly ground black pepper

For the tomato salsa
1 tomato, deseeded and diced
a few drops of balsamic vinegar
juice of ½ lime
pinch of dried chilli flakes
handful of fresh rocket

1. Scoop out the avocado flesh into a bowl. Mash with the yogurt and lime juice, and season to taste with salt and pepper.

2. In a separate bowl, mix together the tomato salsa ingredients and set aside.

3. Preheat the overhead grill to high. Lightly toast the bread on one side, then lightly spray the untoasted side with oil and grill for 2–3 minutes until crisp and golden.

4. Spread the mashed avocado over the plain grilled side of the bread and top with the smoked salmon. Sprinkle with the tomato salsa and serve.

ALTERNATIVE TOPPINGS
· roasted or grilled red and yellow peppers, aubergine and courgettes, sprinkled with herbs
· hummus, grated carrot, rocket and baby plum tomatoes
· tzatziki, diced cherry tomatoes, black olives and feta
· mashed avocado topped with canned refried beans
· green pesto, diced tomato and mozzarella

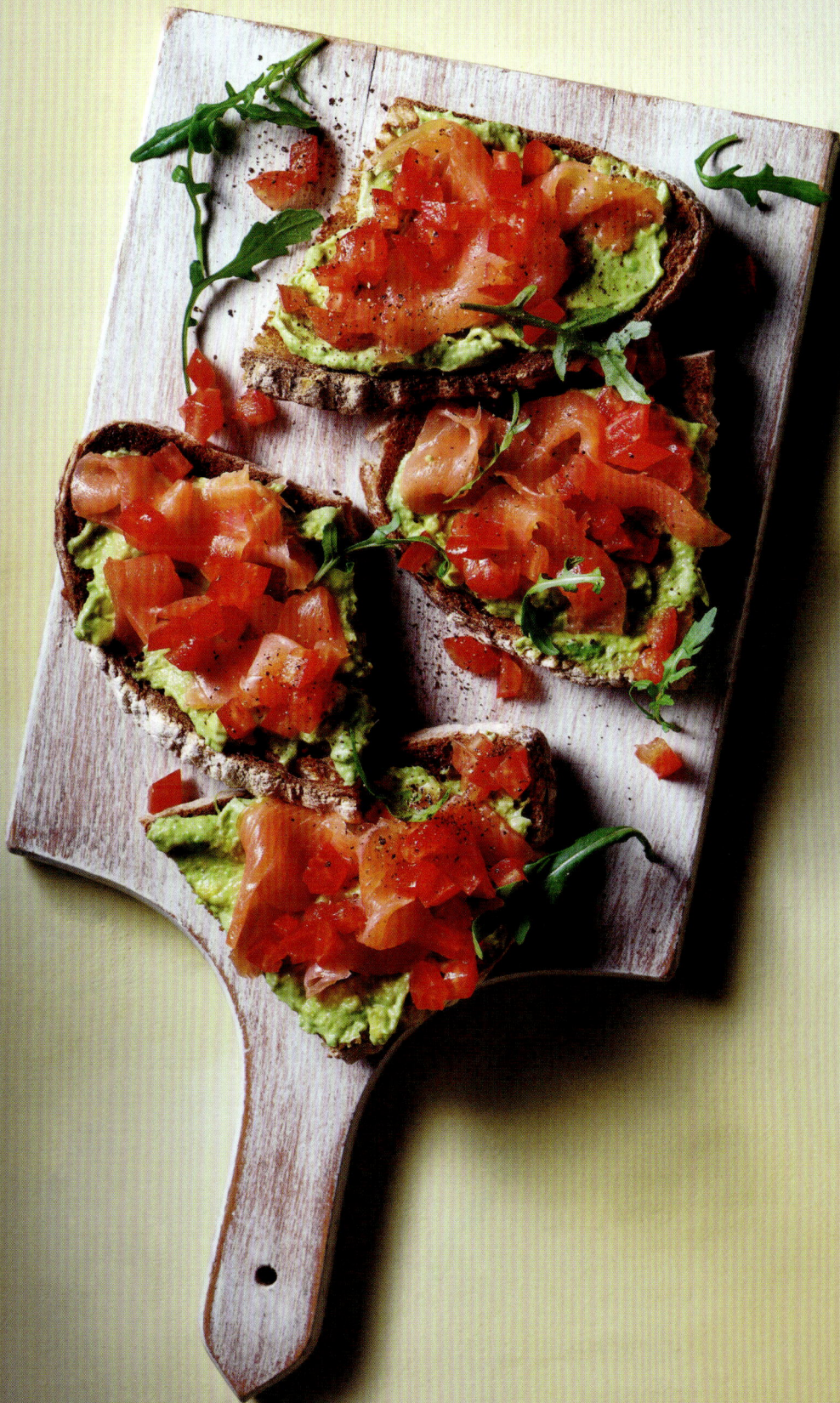

PRAWN & AVOCADO WRAPS

These nutritious wraps are just the thing for when you're feeling peckish and need a quick and healthy snack. They taste delicious and are ready in minutes. You can use up the leftover mango and avocado in a salad.

SERVES
2

PREP
10
minutes

140
kcals
PER SERVING

½ ripe mango, peeled, stoned and diced
½ small avocado, peeled, stoned and diced
100g cooked peeled prawns
a few flat-leaf parsley or coriander sprigs, chopped

1 tbsp fat-free Greek yogurt
grated zest and juice of ½ lime
pinch of cayenne pepper
4 medium little gem lettuce leaves
sea salt and freshly ground black pepper

1. Combine the mango, avocado, prawns and herbs in a bowl.

2. In a separate bowl, mix the yogurt with the lime zest and juice, then gently stir into the prawn and avocado mixture. Season lightly with salt and pepper, if wished, and add a pinch of cayenne.

3. Place the lettuce leaves on a clean surface and divide the prawn-and-avocado mixture between them.

4. Fold the sides of the lettuce leaves over the filling into the centre, and then fold the ends over to make two neat parcels. Turn them over and place, seam-side down, on two plates. Or, if you prefer, just roll up the leaves around the filling. Serve immediately and enjoy!

Tip
Spice up the wraps with a drizzle of sweet chilli sauce.

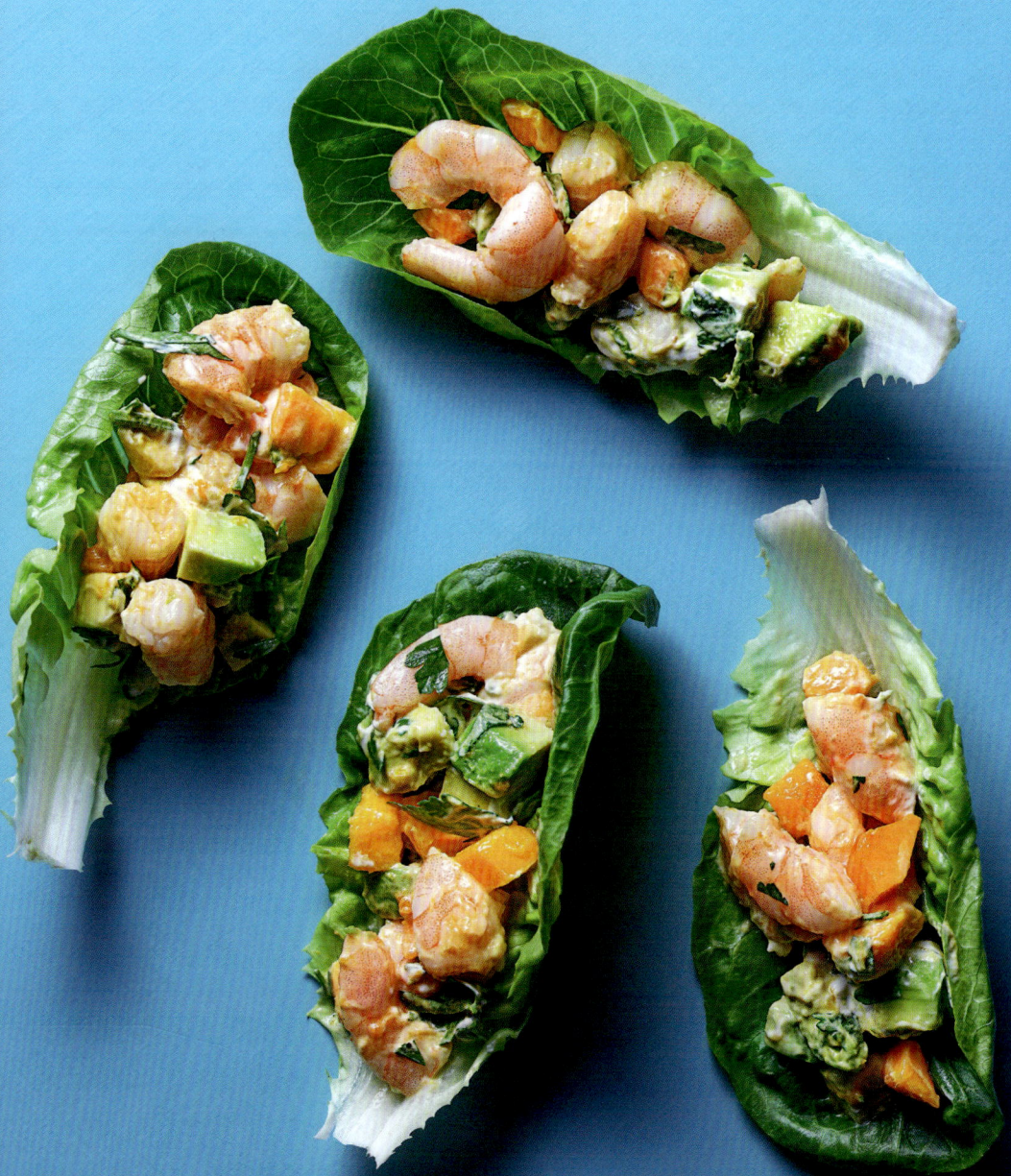

CHUNKY YOGURT DIP

Rustle up this delicious chunky dip and store in an airtight container in the fridge. It keeps well for 2–3 days. It's such a healthy and versatile snack; you can eat it with griddled or raw vegetable crudités, toasted sourdough or wholegrain bread, or even oat cakes, buckwheat crackers and rice cakes.

SERVES
4

PREP
10
minutes

COOK
20–25
minutes

150
kcals
PER SERVING
(DIP ONLY)

400g can chickpeas, rinsed and drained
200g baby plum tomatoes
3 whole garlic cloves, unpeeled
2 tsp olive oil
200g fat-free Greek yogurt
handful of flat-leaf parsley, chopped
sea salt and freshly ground black pepper

To serve
raw or griddled vegetable dippers, such as peppers, courgettes, celery, cucumber, carrots or aubergine slices

1. Preheat the oven to 180°C (gas mark 4).

2. Put the chickpeas, tomatoes and garlic cloves into a baking dish and toss in the olive oil. Season lightly with salt and add a good grinding of black pepper.

3. Bake for 20–25 minutes, or until the tomatoes and garlic have softened.

4. Slip the garlic cloves out of their skins and add them to a bowl with the Greek yogurt. Add most of the parsley and stir to combine, then gently swirl in the chickpeas and softened tomatoes. Sprinkle with the remaining parsley.

5. Serve as a dip with raw or griddled vegetables.

Tip
Make it spicy by swirling in some hot sauce or a dash of harissa.

AIR-FRIED SWEET POTATO CRISPS

For a movie-night treat, you can't beat a bowl of these delicious homemade air-fried sweet potato crisps. Healthier and lower in calories than any you can buy, these crisps skip the deep-frying process, reducing the amount of fat without compromising on flavour. Sweet potatoes are fibre-rich and full of antioxidants. They crisp up to a naturally sweet treat in an air fryer, and because you're in control of the ingredients, you can avoid the excess salt and preservatives often found in supermarket versions.

SERVES
6

450g sweet potatoes
2 tsp cornflour
1 tbsp olive oil

½–1 tsp sea salt
1 tsp smoked paprika
freshly ground black pepper

PREP
15
minutes

1. Wash and peel the sweet potatoes before slicing them as thinly as possible. This is best done with a mandoline, if you have one. Pat dry with kitchen paper to remove excess moisture.

2. Soak the slices in cold water for 30 minutes, then pat dry with kitchen paper once more. Soaking removes the starch and makes the crisps even crisper.

SOAK
30
minutes

3. Transfer the slices to a bowl and dust with the cornflour, tossing gently to evenly coat.

4. Drizzle over the olive oil and then sprinkle with the sea salt, smoked paprika and black pepper. Toss again.

COOK
15–20
minutes

5. Preheat the air fryer to 170°C.

6. Place the sweet potatoes in the air fryer basket in a single layer – you may have to cook them in batches, depending on the size of your air fryer. Cook for 15–20 minutes, shaking the basket at 5-minute intervals, and checking frequently until crisp.

90
kcals
PER SERVING

7. Store in an airtight container at room temperature for up to 3 days.

Tip
You can use beetroot, parsnips, swede or carrots instead of sweet potatoes. These root vegetables will not need soaking before air frying.

SNACKS

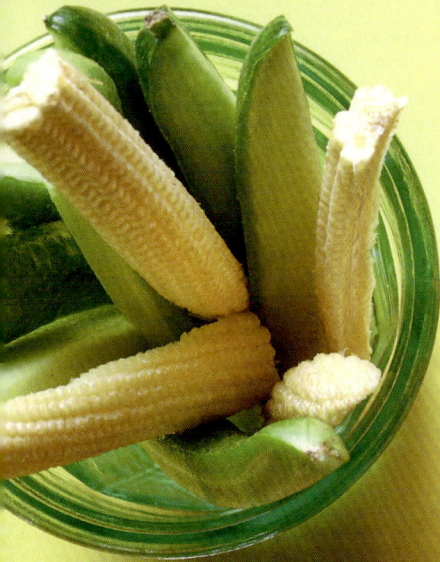

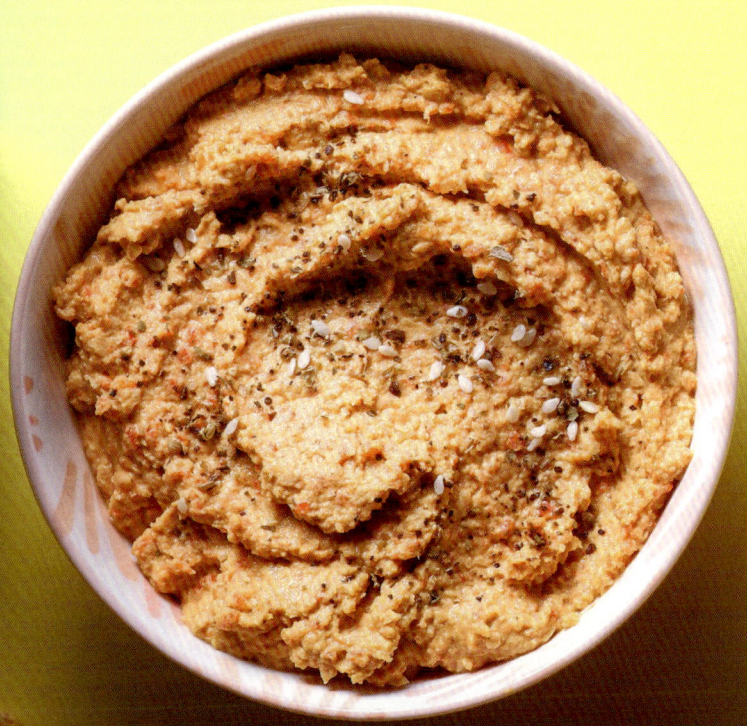

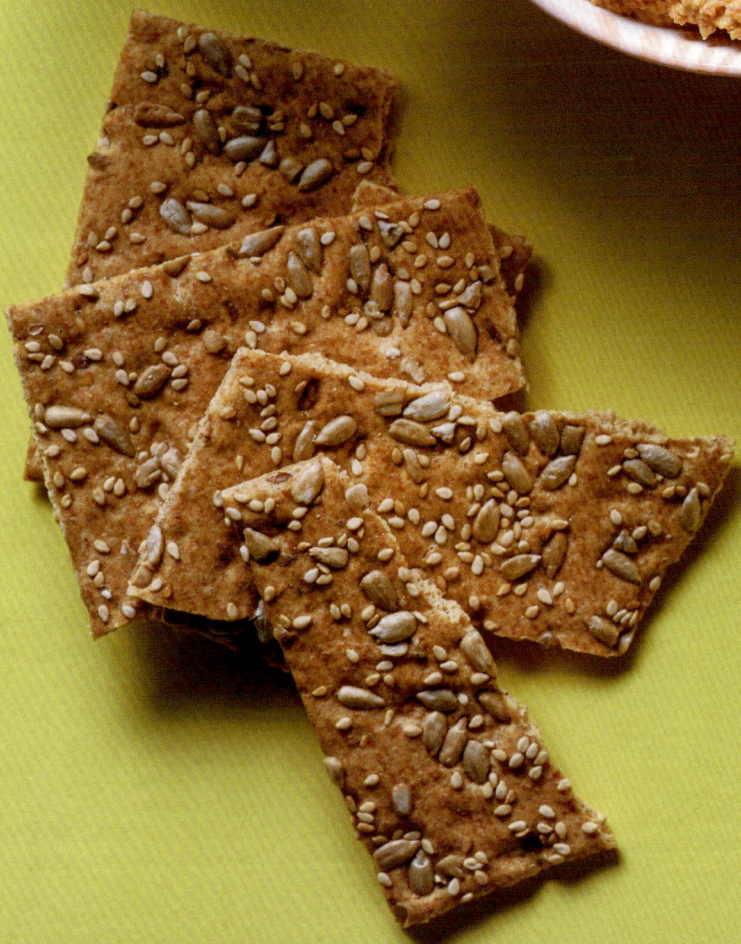

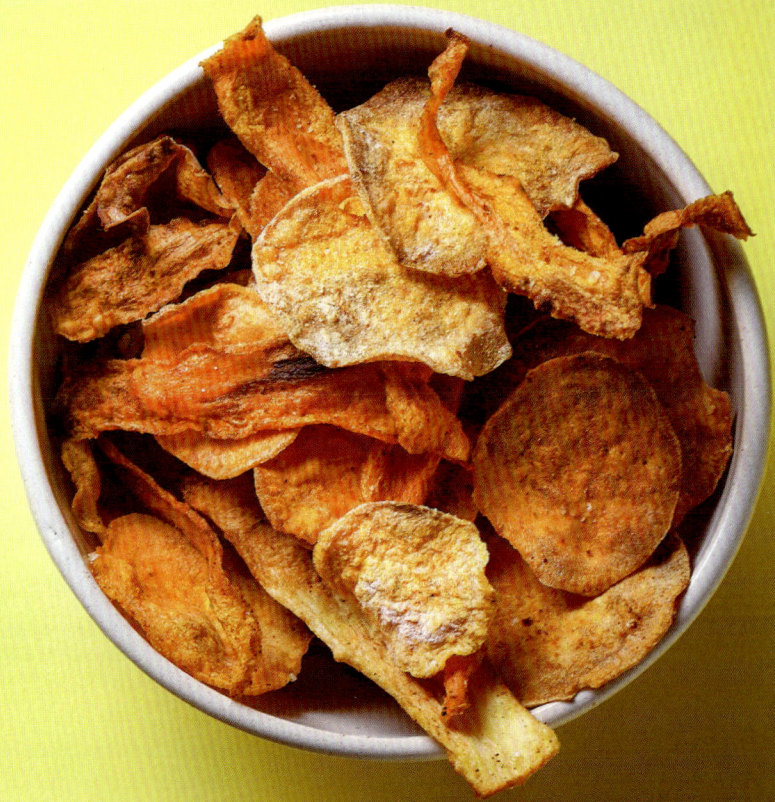

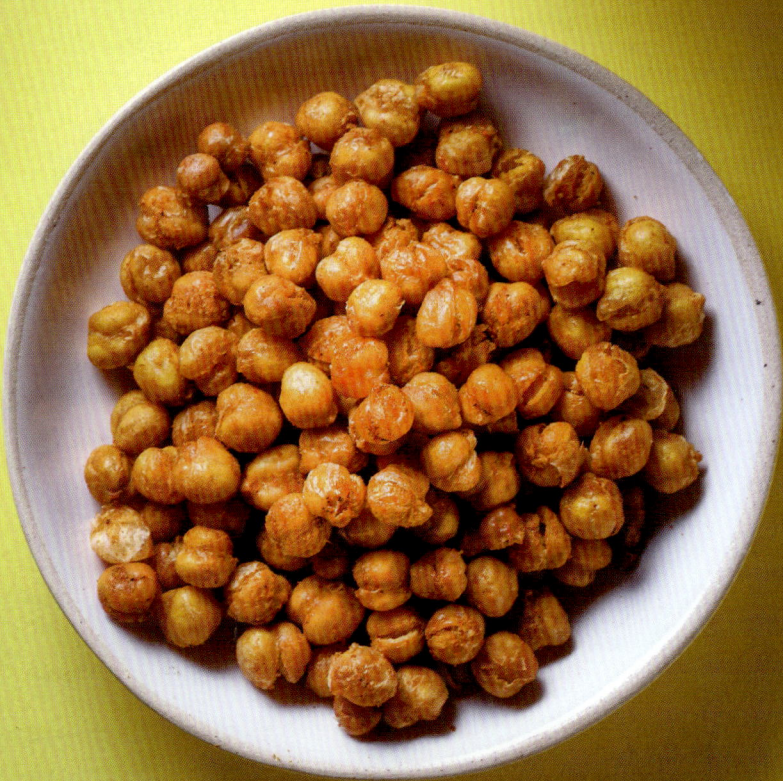

BANANA CHOC ICY POLES

These fabulous frozen banana lollies are a good way of using up leftover ripe bananas. The good news is that bananas, nuts and chocolate all contain fibre. Dark chocolate (over 70 per cent cocoa solids) also contains polyphenols, which fuel the growth of beneficial gut bacteria.

MAKES
8

4 ripe medium bananas
100g dark chocolate chips
   (minimum 70 per cent cocoa
   solids)

½ tsp coconut oil
75g chopped almonds

PREP
15
minutes

1. Peel the bananas and halve horizontally (not lengthways). Insert a lolly stick into the sliced ends and place them side by side on a freezer-proof tray lined with baking parchment. Freeze for at least 10 hours or overnight.

FREEZE
10–11
hours

2. When you're ready to make the icy poles, combine the chocolate chips and coconut oil in a heatproof bowl and melt in the microwave in 30-second bursts, or suspend the bowl over a pan of gently simmering water and stir to melt. As soon as the mixture is melted and glossy, remove from the heat.

175
kcals
PER SERVING

3. Dip a frozen banana into the melted chocolate and then roll in the chopped nuts. Repeat with the remaining bananas and nuts and place them on the lined tray. Return to the freezer for at least 30 minutes. The icy poles will keep well in the freezer for up to 1 week.

Tip
You will need 8 wooden lolly sticks.

FROZEN FRUITY YOGURT CLUSTERS

For a satisfying sweet treat, these frozen fruity yogurt clusters are sure to hit the spot! Not only are they delicious, but they also come loaded with health benefits. The tangy yogurt brings a probiotic boost to your gut, while the fresh berries are packed with antioxidants. We've topped them off with dark chocolate for a fibre-rich crunchy bite.

MAKES
8

PREP
20
minutes

FREEZE
OVERNIGHT
+30 minutes

105
kcals
PER SERVING

200g fresh berries, such as
 blueberries, raspberries or
 strawberries
150g fat-free Greek yogurt

1 tsp runny honey
100g dark chocolate chips
 (minimum 70 per cent cocoa
 solids)

1. Combine the berries in a bowl – if using strawberries, chop them into smaller pieces first. Gently stir in the yogurt and honey, making sure the berries are evenly distributed throughout the mixture.

2. Drop small spoonfuls of the fruit-and-yogurt mixture on to a freezer-proof tray lined with baking parchment. You should end up with 8 dollops. Freeze overnight.

3. The following day, melt the chocolate chips into a heatproof bowl and melt in the microwave in 30-second bursts, or suspend the bowl over a pan of gently simmering water and stir to melt. As soon as they melt, remove from the heat.

4. Quickly dip the frozen fruity yogurt clusters into the melted chocolate, then place them back on the lined tray. Return to the freezer for at least 30 minutes. The clusters will keep well in the freezer for up to 3 weeks.

Tip
Try coating the clusters with chopped hazelnuts after dipping them into the melted chocolate.

SNACKS

dinners

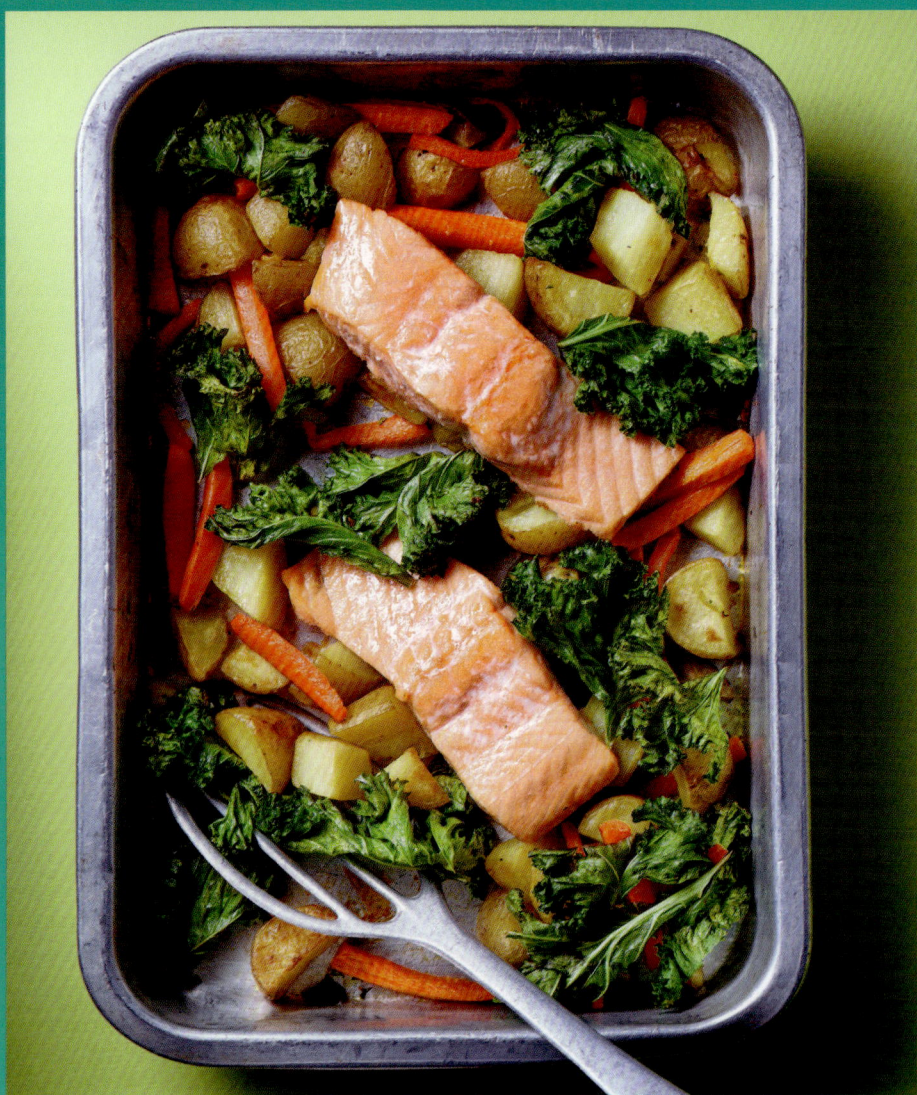

SALMON & CRISPY POTATO TRAYBAKE

Sweet and citrusy, this salmon traybake is so delicious. Roasted carrots naturally caramelise when cooked, while the zesty lemon yogurt balances the flavours beautifully. Salmon is not just a heart-healthy fish, but is also loaded with gut-loving nutrients that can help improve digestion. We've added dark green leafy kale, which turns crispy in the oven and is packed with antioxidants to keep your insides in tiptop shape.

SERVES
2

PREP
10
minutes

COOK
25
minutes

410
kcals
PER SERVING

300g new potatoes, cut into small chunks
2 carrots, peeled and cut into matchsticks
2 tsp olive oil
100g curly kale, stalks removed, roughly chopped
pinch of dried chilli flakes
2 skinless salmon fillets (about 100g each)

4 tbsp fat-free Greek yogurt
grated zest of 1 lemon
a few mint or flat-leaf parsley sprigs, chopped
sea salt and freshly ground black pepper
lemon wedges, for squeezing

1. Preheat the oven to 220°C (gas mark 7).

2. Toss the potatoes and carrots in a bowl with 1 teaspoon of the oil until glistening all over. Season with salt and pepper, then tip into a roasting tray, spreading out into an even layer. Bake for 15 minutes, or until starting to colour.

3. In a bowl, massage the remaining oil into the kale, along with the chilli flakes. After the carrots and potatoes have been roasting for 15 minutes, add the kale to the roasting tray and stir to combine. Then add the salmon fillets, turning them in the oily pan juices. Return the tray to the oven and bake for another 10 minutes, or until the salmon is cooked through and opaque. Check the seasoning, adding more salt and pepper if liked.

4. Meanwhile, in a bowl, mix the yogurt with the lemon zest and chopped herbs.

5. Serve the roasted vegetables and salmon with the herby yogurt and lemon wedges for squeezing.

Tip
You can cook firm white fish fillets in the same way.

PAN-SEARED TUNA
with Mediterranean vegetables

It's the combination of capers, olives, chili flakes, garlic and onion that really bring the full flavours of the Med to this tasty pan-seared tuna. Season your tuna generously and sear it quickly on each side to maintain the juicy flavours.

SERVES
2

PREP
10
minutes

COOK
20
minutes

390
kcals
PER SERVING

olive oil spray
1 onion, diced
1 red or yellow pepper, cut into chunks
2 garlic cloves, crushed
400g can chopped or cherry tomatoes
1 tbsp capers
8 black olives, stoned
pinch of red pepper flakes or dried chilli flakes

200g canned white beans, rinsed and drained
2 fresh tuna steaks (about 100g each)
a few flat-leaf parsley or basil sprigs, chopped
juice of ½ lemon
80g broccoli or cauliflower florets
basil sprigs, to serve
sea salt and freshly ground black pepper

1. Lightly spray a frying pan or sauté pan with oil and set over a low–medium heat. Add the onion and red or yellow pepper and cook, stirring occasionally, for 5 minutes, or until softened. Stir in the garlic and cook for 2 minutes more.

2. Add the tomatoes, capers, olives and red pepper or chilli flakes. Increase the heat to medium and cook for 5 minutes, then stir in the beans.

3. Push the bean-and-tomato mixture aside and place the tuna steaks in the centre of the pan. Cover with a lid and cook for 4 minutes, then turn the steaks and cook, uncovered, for 3–4 minutes. Gently stir the herbs and lemon juice into the bean and tomato mixture.

4. Meanwhile, cook the broccoli or cauliflower in a pan of boiling salted water until just tender. Drain well.

5. Place a steak on each plate and spoon the tomato-and-bean mixture over the top. Garnish with basil and serve with the broccoli.

Tip
If you can't get fresh tuna, use canned tuna chunks in spring water instead.

VIETNAMESE SALMON NOODLE BOWL

This salmon dish is bursting with flavour and full of heart-healthy goodness. The delicious marinade is a blend of gut-friendly ingredients with a hint of sugar for a perfectly balanced taste. We've added pak choi, a type of Chinese cabbage, for a crunchy bite. If you can't find it, just steam some spring greens, kale, spinach or dark green cabbage.

SERVES
2

PREP
15
minutes

MARINATE
30
minutes

COOK
10
minutes

400
kcals
PER SERVING

2 skinless salmon fillets (about 100g each)
olive oil spray
80g vermicelli rice noodles (dry weight)
1 tsp nam pla (fish sauce)
juice of ½ lime
1 red bird's-eye chilli, finely sliced
2 spring onions, finely sliced
2 heads of pak choi, halved lengthways

1 tsp toasted sesame seeds
2 tsp sweet chilli sauce (optional)

For the marinade
1 tbsp nam pla (fish sauce)
1 tbsp light soy sauce
1 tsp lemon juice
2cm piece of fresh root ginger, peeled and grated
1 garlic clove, crushed
1 tsp light brown sugar

1. Whisk together all the marinade ingredients in a shallow dish. Add the salmon fillets and turn them in the marinade until coated all over. Cover with cling film and chill in the fridge for 30 minutes.

2. Lightly spray a griddle pan with oil and set over a medium–high heat. When the pan is hot, add the salmon fillets and cook for 3–4 minutes on each side, or until cooked right through.

3. Meanwhile, cook the vermicelli noodles according to the instructions on the packet. Drain well and toss in a large bowl with the nam pla, lime juice, chilli and spring onions.

4. Bring a pan of water to the boil, then reduce the heat to medium. Steam the pak choi in a covered basket over the pan for 3–5 minutes.

5. Divide the noodles between plates and top with the salmon. Sprinkle with sesame seeds and serve with the pak choi and a drizzle of sweet chilli sauce.

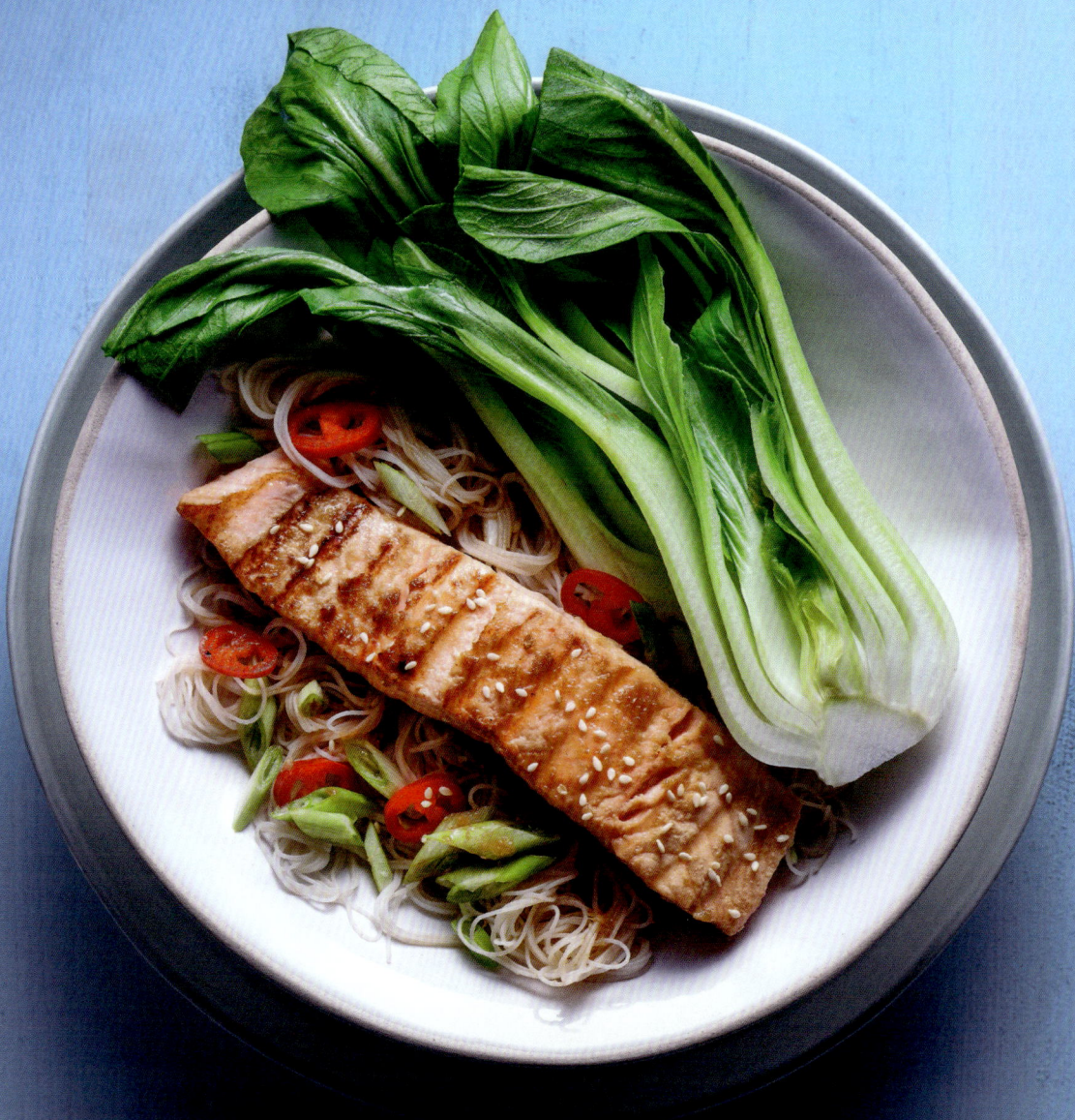

Tip

The salmon also tastes delicious cooked over hot coals or charcoal on a barbecue. Alternatively, you can bake it in the oven at 180°C (gas mark 4) for 20 minutes.

JAPANESE COD
with stir-fry greens

This dinner combines delicious Japanese flavours with crisp Asian greens. The secret to this slimming-friendly dish lies in marinating the cod overnight, giving it time to absorb all those gorgeous umami flavours. The following evening, a heart-healthy, nutritious dinner is ready in just 20 minutes.

SERVES
2

PREP
15
minutes

MARINATE
OVERNIGHT

COOK
30
minutes

370
kcals
PER SERVING

2 x 150g boned and skinned thick cod fillets
60g brown rice (dry weight)
olive oil spray
2cm piece fresh root ginger, peeled and shredded
2 garlic cloves, finely sliced
1 red chilli, shredded
2 spring onions, shredded
200g spring greens, pak choi or spinach, shredded
2 tsp light soy sauce

For the marinade
2 tbsp sake (Japanese rice wine)
2 tbsp mirin
1 tsp runny honey
2 tbsp white miso paste

1. Make the marinade: put the sake, mirin and honey in a pan and set over a high heat. Stir gently until it comes to a boil, then reduce the heat to low and add the miso. Stir until it dissolves and take the pan from the heat. Leave to cool.

2. Pour into a container and add the cod fillets. Turn them in the marinade until they are coated all over. Cover and marinate in the fridge overnight.

3. The following day, cook the brown rice according to the instructions on the packet.

4. Meanwhile remove the cod from the marinade and pat dry with kitchen paper. Lightly spray a frying pan with oil and set over a medium–high heat. Add the fillets to the hot pan and cook for 2–3 minutes, until browned underneath. Turn them over and cook for 2–3 minutes.

Tip

For a Japanese touch, serve the cod sprinkled with 1 tsp white sesame seeds with some pickled ginger on the side.

5. Place the pan under a preheated overhead grill and cook for 5–10 minutes, or until the cod is flaky and cooked right through.

6. Meanwhile, spray a clean pan with oil and set over a medium–high heat. Stir-fry the ginger, garlic and chilli for 2 minutes. Add the spring onions, greens and soy sauce and stir-fry for 2 minutes.

7. Serve the cod immediately with the stir-fried greens and brown rice.

NOTES

It's the savoury and very distinctive umami flavours that make this dinner so delicious. Miso is made from fermented soybean paste and even just a spoonful can make all the difference to a marinade or broth. Like soy sauce, another Japanese umami ingredient, it is quite salty with a concentrated taste, so you don't need to use much of it. The fermentation process means it's good for your gut biome as it provides beneficial bacteria.

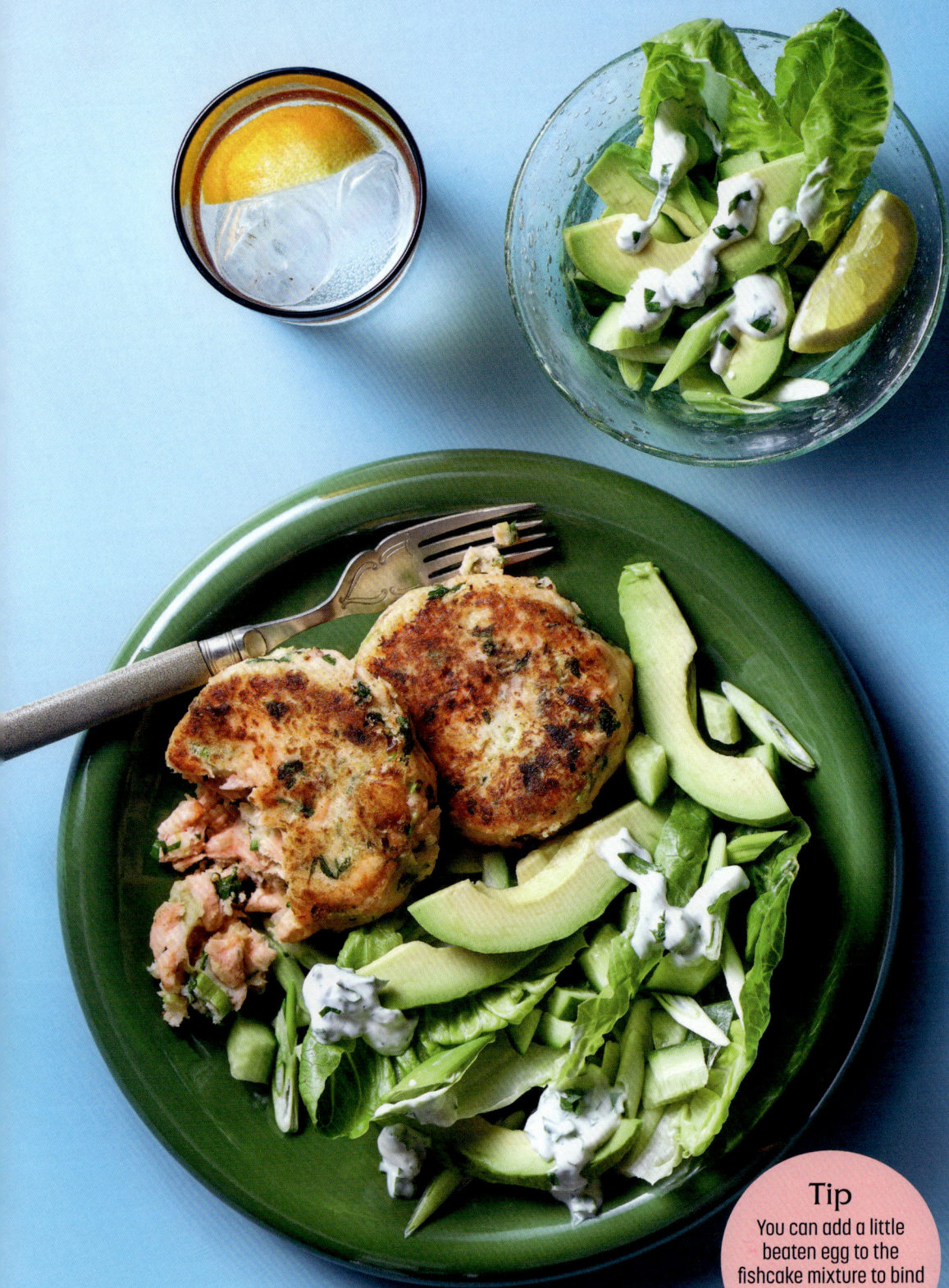

Tip
You can add a little beaten egg to the fishcake mixture to bind it and make it stiffer.

SALMON FISHCAKES & GREEN GODDESS SALAD

These fishcakes are a fantastically healthy, slimming-friendly, and full of omega-3 fatty acids. They're real comfort food and make a very healthy and economical dinner, especially if you use leftover salmon or even canned. You can prepare the fishcakes in advance and chill in the fridge for up to 24 hours to cook later.

SERVES
2

PREP
15
minutes

CHILL
30
minutes

COOK
25
minutes

410
kcals
PER SERVING

225g potatoes, peeled and cut into large chunks
2 tbsp fat-free Greek yogurt
175g cooked salmon fillets
2 spring onions, finely chopped
4 tbsp chopped flat-leaf parsley
a few chives, snipped
1 tsp capers, chopped
½ tsp cayenne pepper
grated zest of ½ lemon and 2 tsp juice
1 tbsp plain flour

olive oil spray
sea salt and freshly ground black pepper
lemon wedges, to serve

For the green goddess salad
handful of crisp lettuce leaves
2 spring onions, sliced
¼ cucumber, diced
1 small avocado, peeled, stoned and cubed
1 quantity green goddess dressing (see page 84)

1. Cook the potatoes in a pan of salted boiling water for 15 minutes, or until just tender. Drain and mash until smooth, then stir in the yogurt.

2. Break the salmon into large flakes and add to the mashed potato, along with the spring onions, herbs, capers, cayenne and lemon zest and juice. Season with salt and pepper. Shape the mixture into four patties. Dust with the flour, then cover and chill in the fridge for 30 minutes.

3. Lightly spray a frying pan with oil and place over a medium heat. Add the fishcakes and cook for 4 minutes on each side until golden brown.

4. To make the salad, combine the lettuce, spring onions, cucumber and avocado in a bowl. Pour over the dressing and toss lightly.

5. Serve the fish cakes with the salad, with some lemon wedges on the side for squeezing.

BAKED HADDOCK with Bombay-style potatoes

This is a wonderful dish, full of flavours and all the goodness that fresh haddock brings, such as omega-3 fatty acids. The Bombay potatoes are super easy to make, and add a kick of spice and goodness for your gut.

SERVES
2

PREP
15
minutes

CHILL
30
minutes

COOK
30–35
minutes

320
kcals
PER SERVING

juice of ½ lime
1 tsp curry paste
1 tsp grated fresh root ginger
4 tbsp fat-free Greek yogurt
2 skinless haddock fillets (about 150g each)

For the Bombay-style potatoes
300g potatoes, peeled and cubed
½ tsp ground cumin
¼ tsp ground coriander

good pinch of ground turmeric
a few coriander sprigs, chopped
sea salt and freshly ground black pepper

For the garlicky greens
olive oil spray
2 garlic cloves, crushed
1 red chilli, deseeded and finely sliced
150g spring greens, green cabbage or kale, finely sliced

1. Combine the lime juice, curry paste, ginger and yogurt in a dish. Coat the haddock fillets in the mixture. Cover with cling film and chill in the fridge for 30 minutes.

2 Preheat the oven to 180°C (gas mark 4) and line a baking dish with foil. Put the haddock into the prepared baking dish and bake for 15 minutes.

4. Meanwhile, cook the potatoes in a pan of lightly salted boiling water for 10–15 minutes until tender. Drain well and stir in the ground spices and chopped coriander. Season to taste with salt and pepper.

5. Lightly spray a wok or large frying pan with oil and set over a medium–high heat. Add the garlic, chilli and greens, and stir-fry for 2–3 minutes.

6. When the haddock is cooked, preheat the overhead grill to high, and pop the baking dish under it for 3–5 minutes until the tops of the haddock fillets are just starting to char.

7. Serve the fish with the spicy potatoes and greens.

Tip
You can use other white fish fillets in this recipe, such as cod or monkfish.

SUPER-SPEEDY PRAWN CURRY

Super speedy, slimming and satisfying! This is as good as it gets – a fabulous spicy prawn curry from start to finish in just 20 minutes. That beats any takeaway! The brown rice, onion, red pepper and spinach, together with the herbs and spices, provide a fibre-rich boost for your gut. Feel free to adjust the spices to suit your tastes. If you like, you can add more veg for extra goodness – frozen peas work brilliantly.

SERVES
2

PREP
5
minutes

COOK
15
minutes

415
kcals
PER SERVING

olive oil spray
1 onion, diced
1 red pepper, diced
2 garlic cloves, crushed
1 tsp cumin seeds
1 tsp grated fresh root ginger
1 tsp ground turmeric
1 tbsp curry paste
200ml canned reduced-fat
    coconut milk
200g canned chopped
    tomatoes

250g frozen raw peeled king
    prawns, defrosted
grated zest of 1 lime or lemon
60g baby spinach leaves
handful of coriander, chopped,
    plus extra for sprinkling
60g brown rice (raw weight)
1 red chilli, finely sliced
    (optional)
sea salt and freshly ground
    black pepper

1. Lightly spray a pan with oil and set over a medium heat. Add the onion, red pepper and garlic and cook, stirring occasionally, for 5 minutes until softened but not coloured. Stir in the cumin seeds, ginger and turmeric and cook for 1 minute, then add the curry paste and cook for 1–2 minutes more.

2. Add the coconut milk and tomatoes, then increase the heat to high and bring to the boil. Once boiling, reduce the heat to low and stir in the prawns. Cook for 5 minutes, or until they turn pink, then add the lime zest, spinach and coriander, and cook for another 2 minutes, or until the spinach wilts. Check the seasoning, adding salt and pepper if needed.

3. Meanwhile, cook the rice according to the instructions on the packet.

4. Serve the curry and rice sprinkled with the chilli (if using) and more coriander.

Tip
If you don't like fresh coriander, substitute basil or parsley.

DINNERS

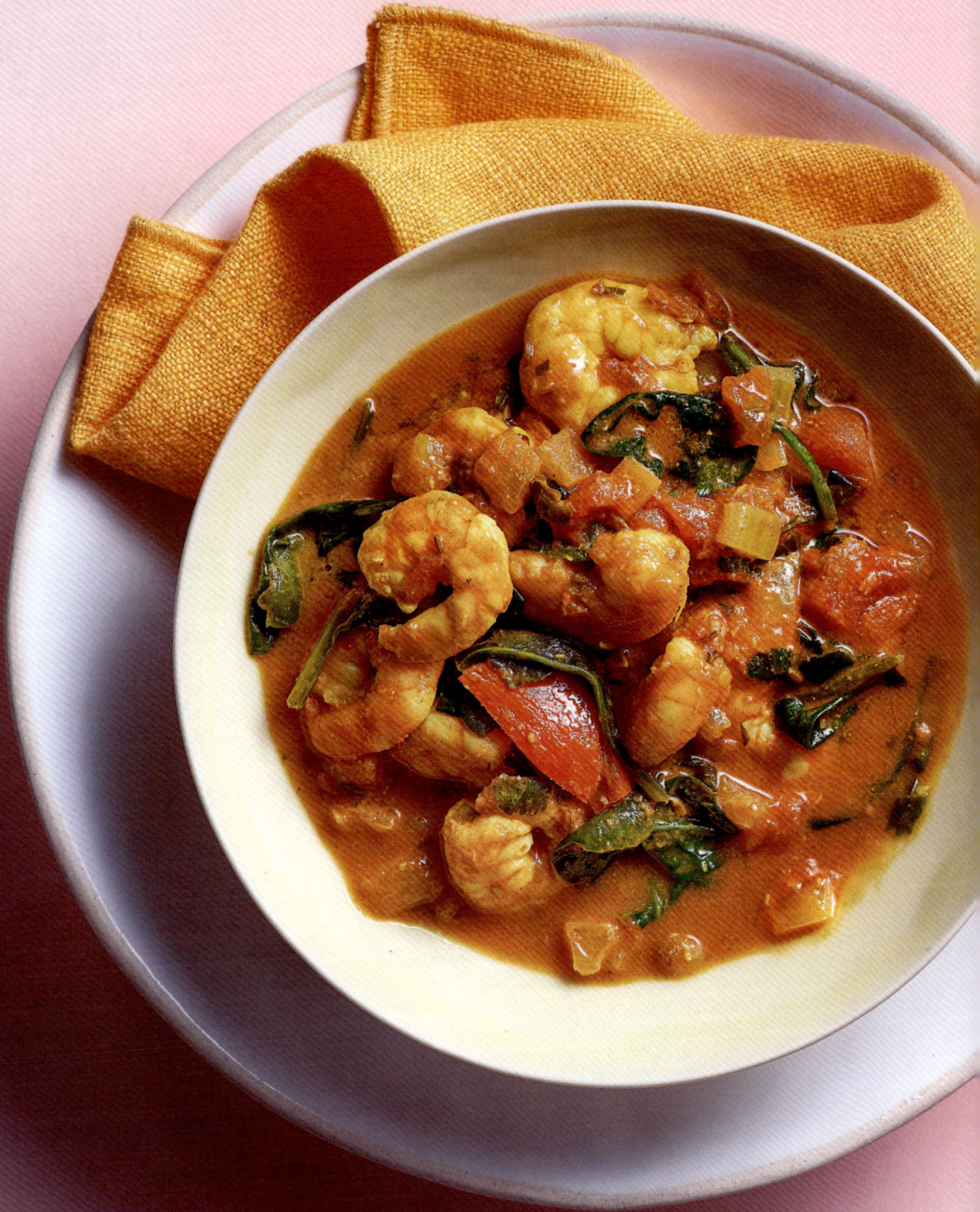

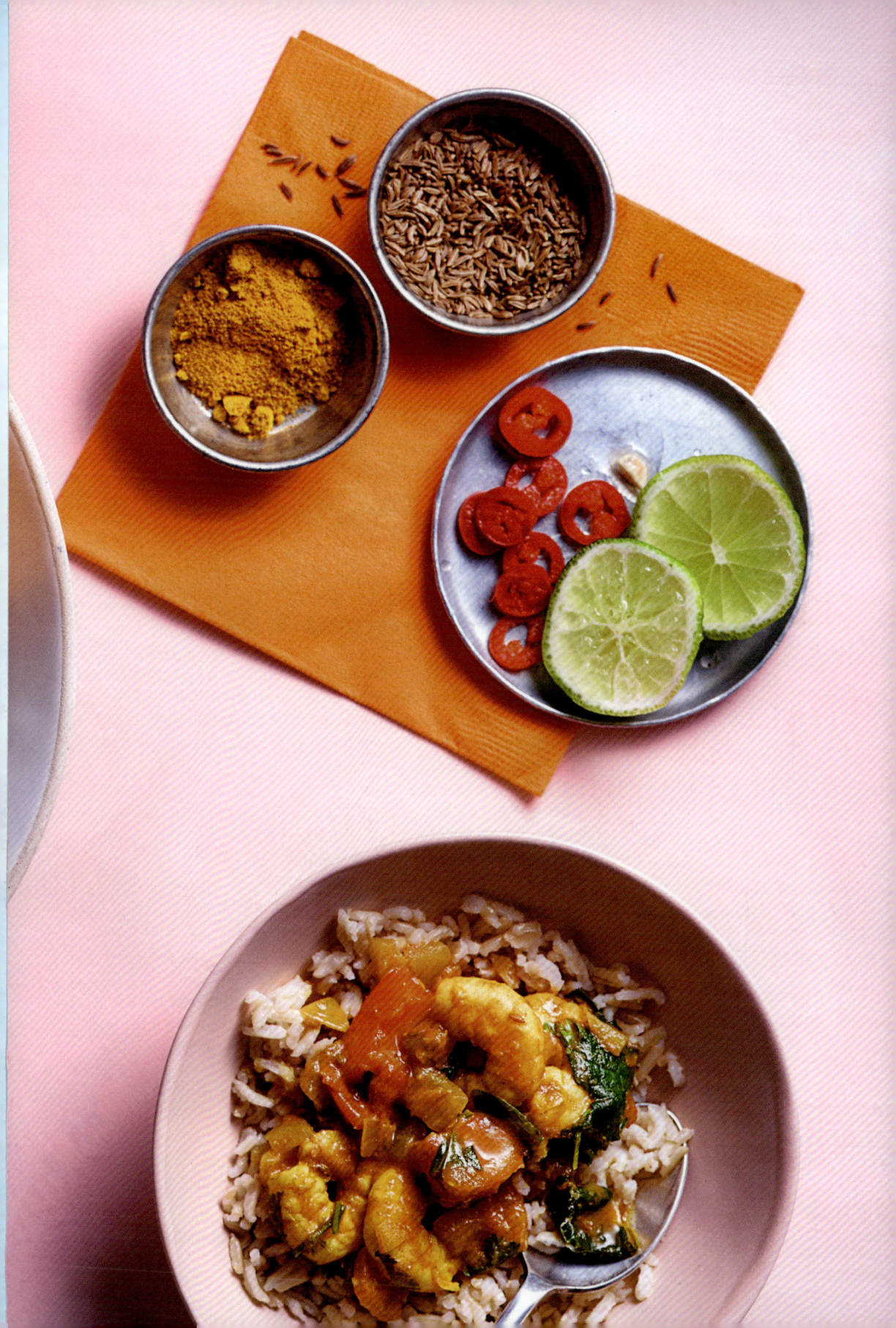

SICILIAN-STYLE SHRIMP SPAGHETTI

If you love garlic, chilli and wine, then you'll adore this pasta dish. A slimming-friendly dinner made with wholewheat spaghetti and simple ingredients, it's like summer on a plate. If you'd like to spice it up even more, add a dash of chilli paste before adding the herbs.

SERVES
2

PREP
5
minutes

COOK
12–15
minutes

370
kcals
PER SERVING

60g wholewheat spaghetti or linguine (dry weight)
olive oil spray
4 garlic cloves, crushed
a good pinch of dried chilli flakes or red pepper flakes
bunch of flat-leaf parsley, finely chopped
bunch of chives, snipped

juice of 1 large lemon
120ml white wine
pinch of caster sugar
2 tomatoes, diced
300g frozen raw peeled king prawns, defrosted
handful of rocket leaves
sea salt and freshly ground black pepper

1. Cook the pasta in a large pan of salted boiling water according to the instructions on the packet. Drain well.

2. Meanwhile, lightly spray a large frying pan with oil and set over a medium heat. Add the garlic and cook for 1 minute without colouring. Stir in the chilli and half of the chopped herbs, then pour in the lemon juice and wine and bring to the boil. Let it bubble away for 5 minutes, or until the liquid reduces and evaporates.

3. Add the sugar, tomatoes and prawns and cook for 2 minutes more, or until the prawns are pink underneath. Flip them over and cook on the other side for 1–2 minutes until pink. Do not overcook, or they will lose their juicy tenderness. Season to taste with salt and pepper, and stir in the remaining herbs.

4. Add the rocket and drained pasta to the pan and gently toss together until everything is lightly coated with the sauce.

5. Divide between two shallow serving bowls and serve immediately.

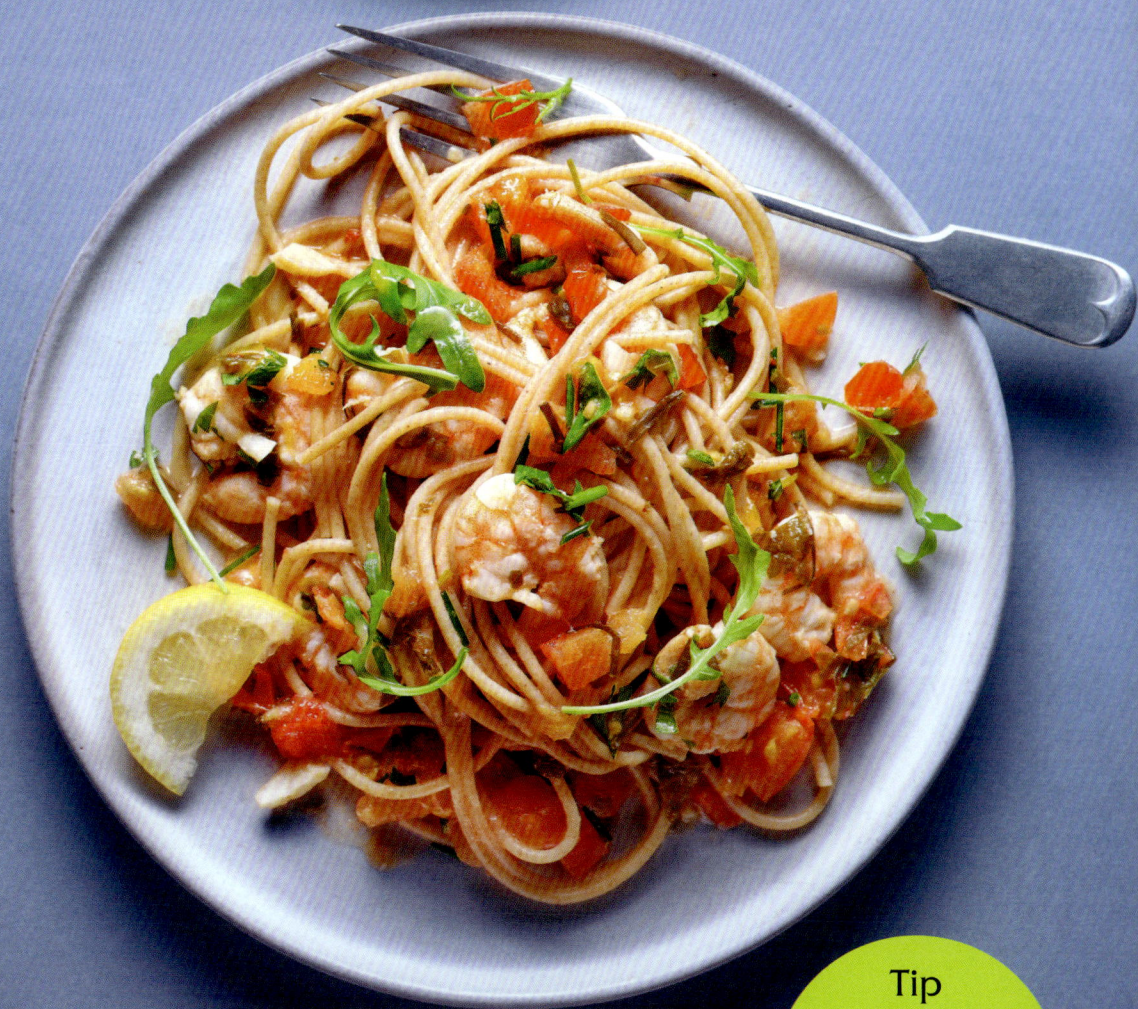

Tip

You can find packs of frozen raw prawns in the freezer aisle in your local supermarket. Be sure to defrost them thoroughly before cooking.

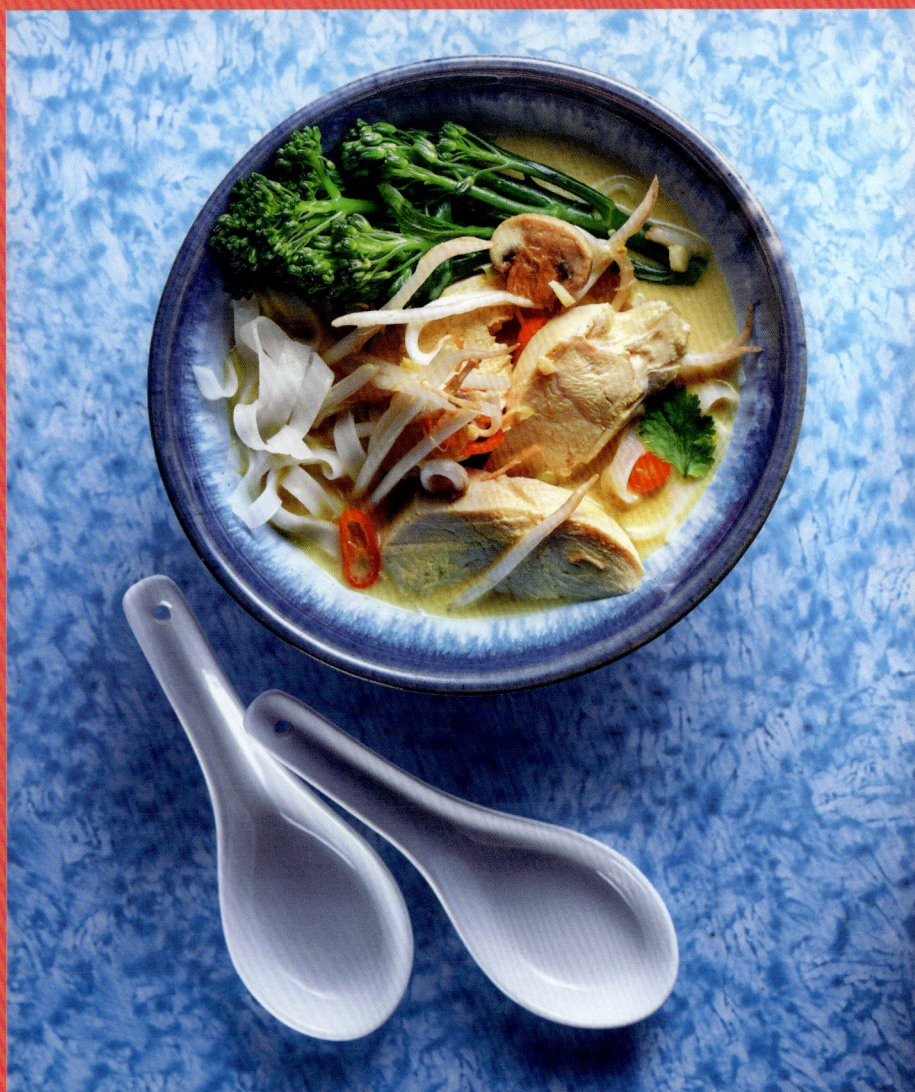

BALSAMIC GLAZED PORK & ROASTED APPLE TRAYBAKE

This fabulously quick and easy glazed pork traybake with sweet roasted apple chunks and vegetables is a comforting, healthy hug for your body. Lean pork is a great source of high-quality protein as well as vitamins B12, B6, niacin and riboflavin, which help reduce stress and fatigue. We've given this dish a nutritious boost with a generous helping of roasted veg, adding more fibre and gut-friendly ingredients.

SERVES
2

PREP
15
minutes

COOK
45–50
minutes

380
kcals
PER SERVING

250g sweet potato, peeled and cut into chunks
2 large carrots, peeled and cut into batons
1 red onion, cut into wedges
100g button mushrooms, halved
a few fresh sage leaves
olive oil spray
1 dessert apple, peeled, cored and cut into chunks

2 lean pork steaks (about 100g each), all visible fat removed
sea salt and freshly ground black pepper

For the balsamic mustard glaze
2 tbsp wholegrain mustard
1 tbsp balsamic vinegar
1 tsp clear honey

1. Preheat the oven to 200°C (gas mark 6).

2. Spread out the sweet potato cubes, carrots, red onion and mushrooms in a roasting tin. Tuck in the sage leaves, season with salt and pepper, and spray lightly with oil. Bake for 20 minutes.

3. Meanwhile, make the balsamic mustard glaze by simply mixing all the ingredients in a bowl.

4. Add the apple pieces and pork steaks to the roasting tin, and drizzle the glaze over the top. Bake for 25–30 minutes, or until the pork steaks are cooked through and the vegetables are tender. Divide between plates and serve.

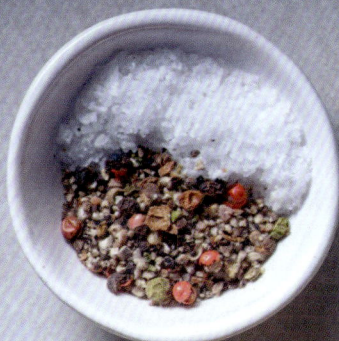

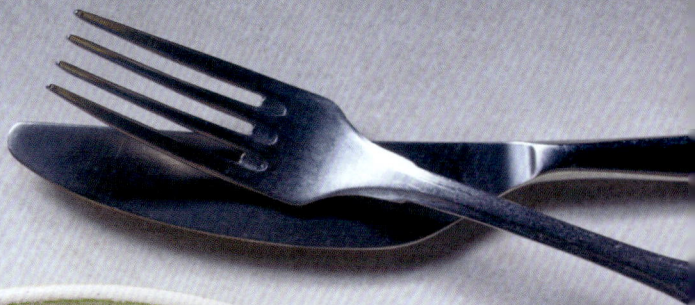

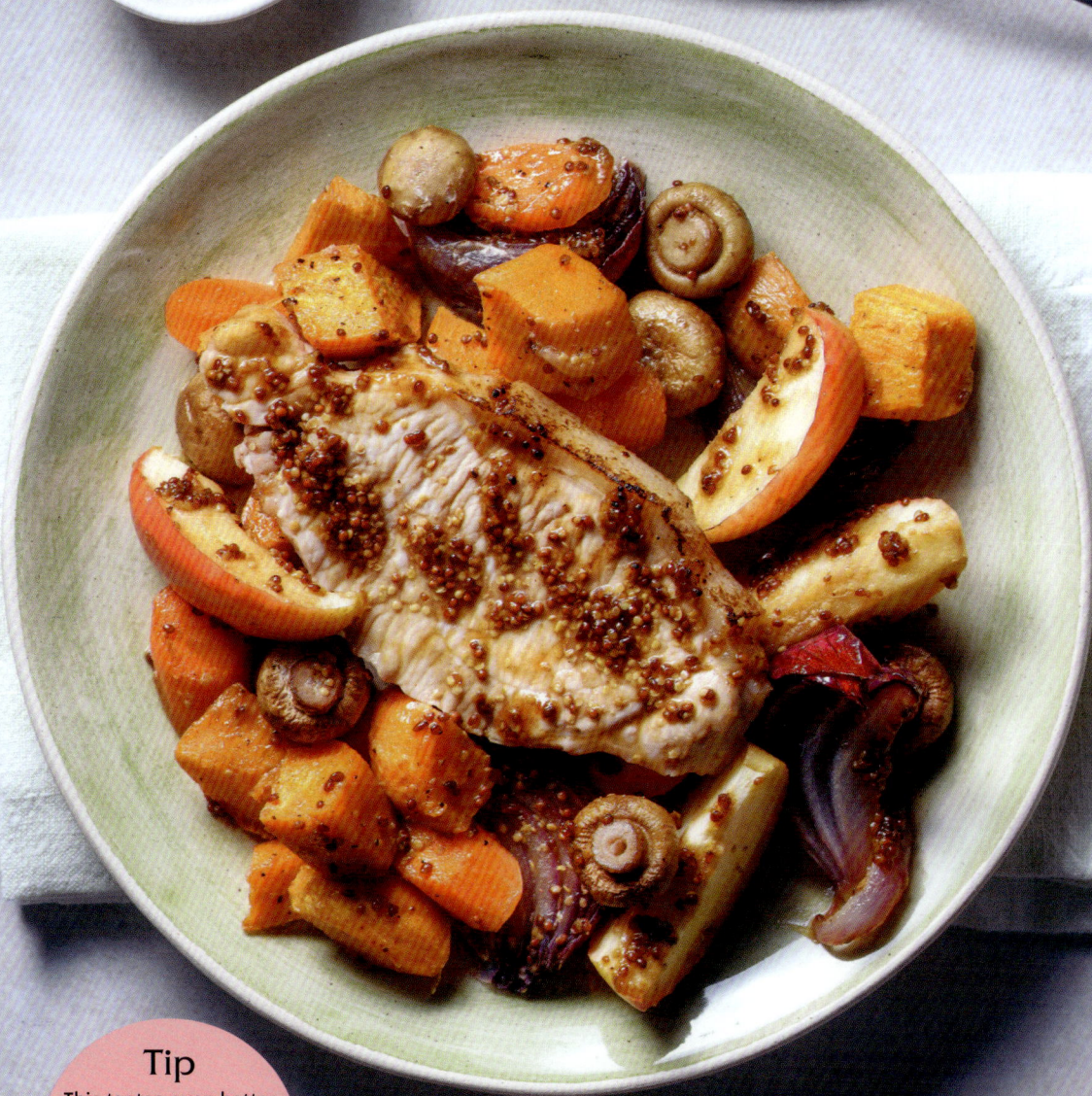

Tip
This tastes even better served with green vegetables, such as broccoli, thin green beans or spinach.

HARISSA-KISSED CHICKEN
with lemon couscous

These North African-inspired harissa-kissed chicken thighs taste utterly delicious paired with zesty lemon couscous. The slimming yet sweet and spicy flavours blend beautifully. You can be creative with the couscous, adding your favourite chopped vegetables, herbs and spices.

SERVES
2

PREP
15
minutes

MARINATE
15
minutes

COOK
12–15
minutes

490
kcals
PER SERVING

1 tsp harissa paste
1 tsp olive oil
1 tsp runny honey
finely grated zest and juice of 1 lemon
4 small skinless bone-in chicken thighs
olive oil spray

For the lemon couscous
60g couscous (dry weight)
finely grated zest and juice of 1 small lemon
100ml hot chicken stock

1 tbsp toasted pine nuts
2 tsp mixed seeds
200g canned chickpeas, rinsed and drained
4 spring onions, chopped
handful of flat-leaf parsley or mint, chopped
sea salt and freshly ground black pepper

For the spiced yogurt
1 tsp harissa paste
60g fat-free Greek yogurt

1. In a bowl, combine the harissa, olive oil, honey, lemon zest and juice. Add the chicken thighs and coat in the mixture. Cover and marinate in the fridge for 15 minutes.

2. Combine the couscous and lemon zest and juice in a heatproof bowl and pour over the hot chicken stock. Stir well, then cover the bowl with a plate and set aside for 10–15 minutes. Once it's ready, fluff up with a fork and stir in the pine nuts, seeds, chickpeas, spring onions and herbs. Season to taste with salt and pepper.

3. Preheat the grill to high. Lightly spray a baking tray with oil, then add the chicken thighs. Cook for 12–15 minutes, turning until cooked right through, sticky and golden brown. Baste once or twice with any leftover marinade.

4. Meanwhile, swirl the harissa paste through the yogurt, then set aside.

5. Serve the chicken immediately with the warm couscous and spiced yogurt.

Tip
For a more aromatic flavour, you could use rose harissa.

HOMEMADE CHICKEN KIEV

Garlicky, buttery and oozing with flavour, we think our oh-so-crispy chicken Kiev is much tastier and lighter than any you'll ever buy readymade. We've amped up the crisp factor by using an air fryer. No air fryer? No problem! We've got you covered with baking instructions too (see note, see page 146). Chicken is a great way to meet your daily protein requirements, and the new potatoes, panko, asparagus, garlic and parsley all provide gut-friendly fibre.

SERVES
2

PREP
20
minutes

FREEZE
15
minutes

COOK
12–15
minutes

410
kcals
PER SERVING

2 skinless chicken breasts (about 125g each)
1 tbsp plain flour
1 small free-range egg, beaten
40g panko breadcrumbs
olive oil spray
200g new potatoes
120g asparagus spears, ends trimmed

a few drops of syrupy balsamic vinegar, for drizzling
sea salt and freshly ground black pepper

For the garlic butter
1 tbsp butter, softened
3 garlic cloves, crushed
2 tbsp chopped flat-leaf parsley

1. To make the garlic butter, combine the butter, garlic and parsley in a bowl and mix well. Shape into a cylinder and wrap tightly in cling film. Freeze for 15 minutes, or until frozen.

2. With a sharp knife, cut a horizontal slit in the side of each chicken breast to make a deep pocket. Cut the frozen garlic butter in half and place one piece in each chicken pocket.

3. Sift the flour into a bowl and season with salt and pepper. Beat the egg in a separate bowl, and tip the breadcrumbs into a third bowl.

4. Dust the chicken breasts with the seasoned flour, shaking off any excess, and then dip them into the beaten egg before rolling them in the breadcrumbs until coated all over.

continues overleaf

4. Preheat the air fryer to 200°C.

5. Lightly spray the coated turkey breasts with oil and place in the air fryer basket, with a little space between them. Cook, turning halfway through, for 8–10 minutes, or until crisp and golden brown and cooked right through. If you insert a meat thermometer, it should read 75°C. Remove from the air fryer and rest for 5 minutes.

6. Serve the turkey Milanese with the red cabbage slaw.

Tip
If red cabbage isn't available, use shredded crispy white or green cabbage instead, and substitute 4 thinly sliced spring onions for the red onion.

NOTES
If you don't have an air fryer, cook the turkey Milanese in a preheated oven at 200°C (gas mark 6) for 15–20 minutes.

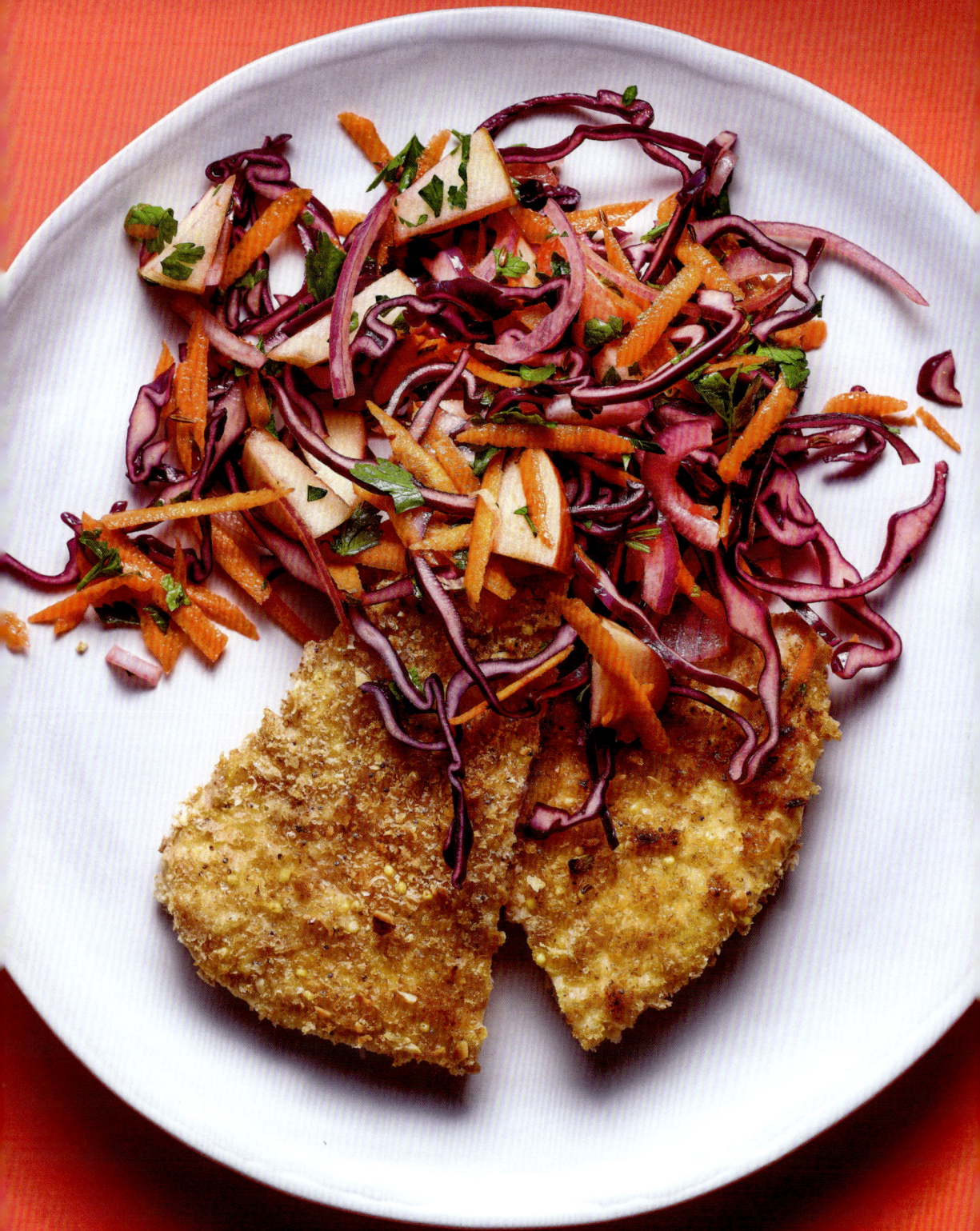

CHICKEN KORMA

A slimming twist on your favourite takeaway, this fragrant chicken korma will fill your kitchen with amazing spicy aromas. We've lowered the calories without compromising on the rich, creamy taste you expect from a korma. We've paired it with a super-tasty tangy red onion chutney, which not only adds flavour but is also full of gut benefits.

SERVES
2

PREP
15
minutes

COOK
25
minutes

370
kcals
PER SERVING

olive oil spray
200g skinless chicken breasts, cut into large chunks
½ red onion, finely sliced
2 garlic cloves, crushed
1 red chilli, diced (see Tip)
1 tsp cumin seeds
2 tsp garam masala
1 tsp ground coriander
1 tsp ground turmeric
1cm piece of fresh root ginger, grated
100ml chicken stock
100ml canned reduced-fat coconut milk

80g fine green beans, trimmed and halved
4 tbsp fat-free Greek yogurt
a few coriander sprigs, chopped
60g basmati rice (dry weight)

For the red onion chutney
½ red onion, finely chopped
1 tsp garam masala
small bunch of coriander, chopped
juice of 1 lime

1. To make the red onion chutney, combine all the ingredients in a small serving bowl. Set aside.

2. Lightly spray a frying pan with oil and set over a medium heat. Add the chicken and onion and cook for 5 minutes, turning occasionally, until the onion is tender and the chicken is golden brown.

3. Add the garlic, chilli and cumin seeds, and cook for 2 minutes, then stir in the ground spices and cook for 2 minutes more. Add the ginger, stock and coconut milk, then bring to the boil. Reduce the heat, cover and simmer for 10 minutes, then add the beans and cook for 5 minutes more, until the chicken is cooked through. Remove from the heat and stir in the yogurt and coriander.

4. Meanwhile, cook the rice according to the instructions on the packet. Divide the korma and rice between two shallow bowls and serve with the chutney.

DINNERS

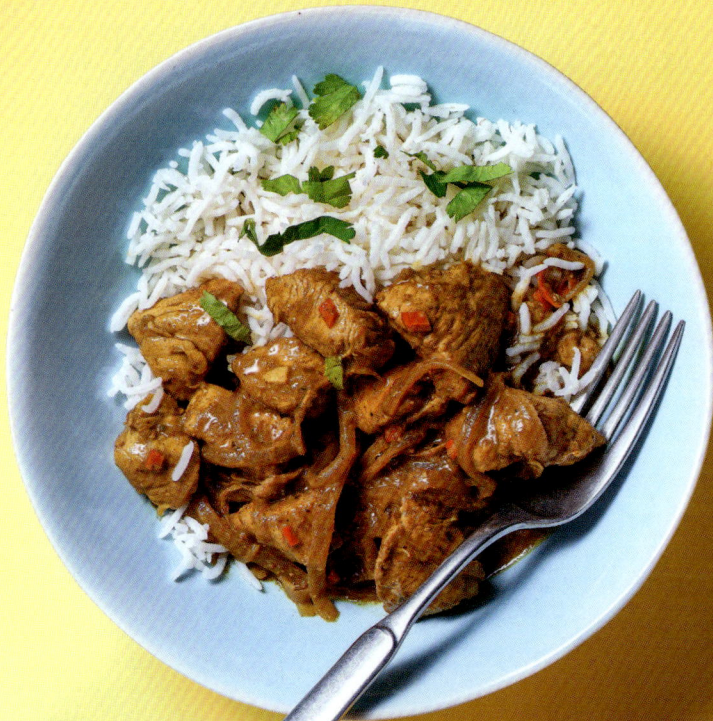

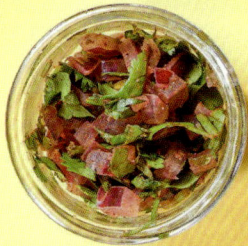

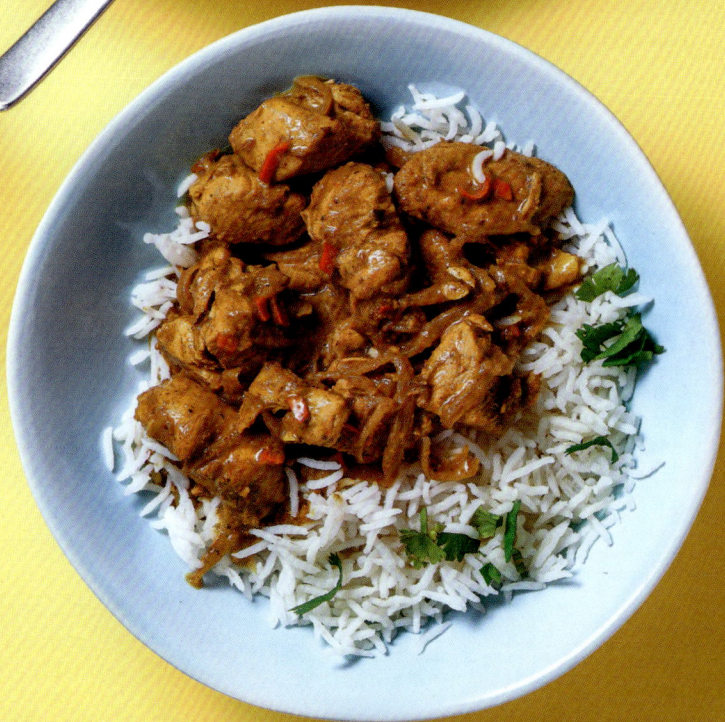

Tip
If you don't have
a fresh chilli, use 1
teaspoon red chilli
powder.

GRIDDLED PIRI PIRI CHICKEN

Bright and vibrant piri piri chicken is always a crowd-pleaser! The spicy marinade is loaded with gut-loving ingredients like paprika, garlic and lemon. Served on a bed of quinoa, which is high in fibre and one of the few 'complete protein' plant-based foods, this dish will help keep your gut happy and your digestion humming along smoothly.

SERVES
2

PREP
10
minutes

MARINATE
2
hours

COOK
15–20
minutes

450
kcals
PER SERVING

2 skinless bone-in chicken legs
olive oil spray
60g quinoa (dry weight)
juice of 1 lime (or ½ lemon)
a few mint, flat-leaf parsley or
    coriander sprigs, chopped
sea salt and freshly ground
    black pepper

For the piri piri marinade
1 tbsp hot chilli sauce
1 tsp smoked paprika
2 garlic cloves, crushed
grated zest and juice of ½
    lemon

1 tsp red wine vinegar
1 tsp olive oil

For the roasted pepper salad
2 red or yellow peppers,
    deseeded and halved
2 tsp olive oil
1 tsp red wine vinegar
1 garlic clove, crushed
pinch of dried oregano
a few basil sprigs

1. Combine all the piri piri marinade ingredients in a bowl. Add the chicken and turn in the marinade until coated all over. Cover and chill in the fridge for at least 2 hours, or overnight if preferred.

2. When you're ready to cook the chicken, lightly spray a griddle pan or non-stick frying pan with oil. Remove the chicken from the marinade and cook over a medium–high heat for 15–20 minutes, turning occasionally, until golden brown and cooked right through. Baste occasionally with any leftover marinade. To check if the chicken is cooked, pierce it with a skewer; the juices should run clear.

3. Meanwhile, cook the quinoa according to the instructions on the packet. When it's cooked, fluff it up with a fork and stir in the citrus juice and herbs. Season to taste.

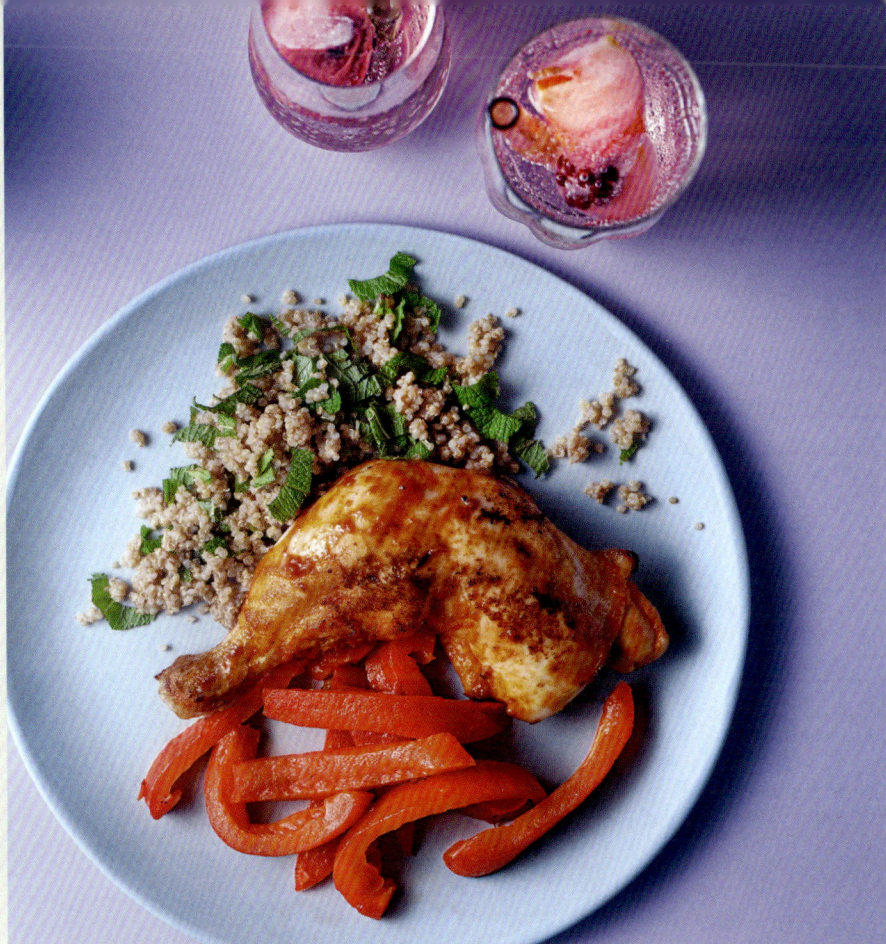

4. Meanwhile make the roasted pepper salad. Grill the peppers under a hot grill for 5–10 minutes until blistered and charred. Alternatively, hold them on a fork over a gas flame. Place in a plastic bag for a few minutes, then peel off the skins and cut the flesh into strips.

5. Blend the oil, vinegar, garlic and oregano to make a dressing and pour it over the warm peppers. Season with salt and pepper, and sprinkle with the basil.

6. Serve the piri piri chicken with the quinoa and roasted pepper salad.

Tip

Chicken wings and breasts can also be marinated and cooked in this way.

TASTY MEATBALLS
with Greek salad

These homemade meatballs are so easy to make, and they taste amazing with our harissa yogurt dip. We've cooked them in an air fryer with a light misting of oil, but if you don't have one, no worries; there are instructions for making them an oven in the tip below. The colourful Greek salad adds a touch of summer to your plate, as well as lots of gut-friendly vegetables.

SERVES
2

PREP
20
minutes

COOK
10–12
minutes

510
kcals
PER SERVING

250g lean minced beef
15g fresh wholemeal breadcrumbs
2 tbsp grated Parmesan cheese
2 garlic cloves, crushed
1 medium free-range egg, beaten
1 small onion, grated
handful of flat-leaf parsley, chopped
a few mint sprigs, chopped
olive oil spray
sea salt and freshly ground black pepper

For the Greek salad
2 juicy tomatoes, cut into chunks
¼ cucumber, cut into chunks
1 green pepper, cubed
¼ red onion, very finely sliced
6 black olives
100g feta cheese, cubed
½ tsp dried oregano
2 tsp fruity olive oil
red wine vinegar, for drizzling

For the harissa yogurt dip
120g fat-free Greek yogurt
1 tsp harissa paste

1. Combine the minced beef, breadcrumbs, Parmesan, garlic, egg, onion and herbs in a bowl. Season with salt and pepper. Stir well, then use your hands to scrunch everything together.

2. Take a small amount of the mixture and, using your hands, roll it into a ball, a little larger than a walnut and smaller than a golf ball. Repeat with the remaining mixture. You should end up with 8–10 meatballs.

3. Preheat the air fryer to 200°C.

4. Lightly spray the meatballs with oil and place them in the air fryer basket in a single layer, leaving a little space between them – you may have to cook them in batches, depending on the size of your air fryer. Cook for 5 minutes, then turn them over and cook for another 5–7 minutes on the other side until browned and cooked right through.

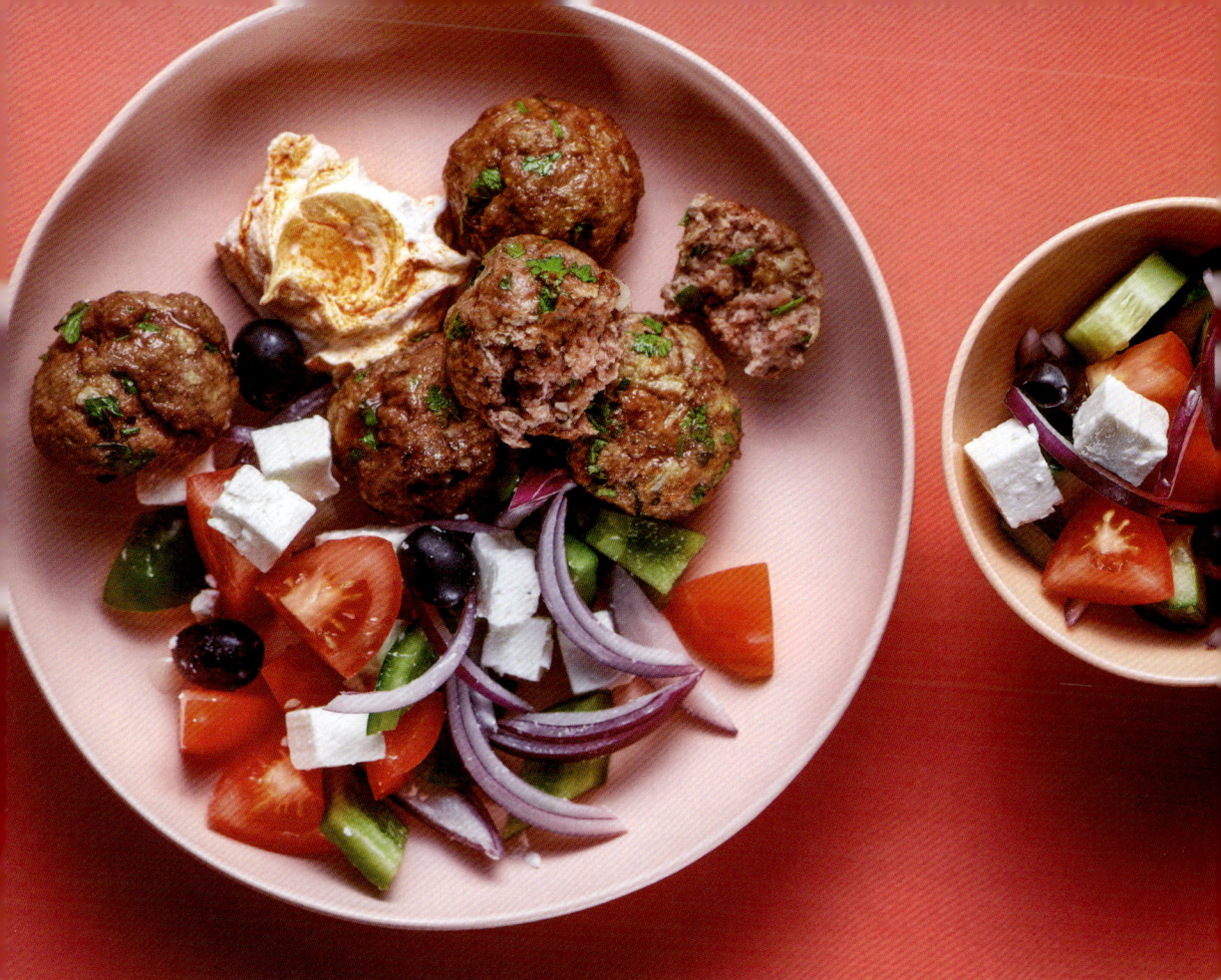

5. Meanwhile, make the Greek salad. Put the vegetables and olives into a bowl and mix well. Top with the feta and sprinkle with oregano. Drizzle with the olive oil and red wine vinegar, and season to taste.

6. To make the harissa yogurt dip, pour the yogurt into a bowl and swirl in the harissa paste. Serve with the meatballs and Greek salad.

Tip

If you don't have an air fryer, bake the meatballs in a preheated oven at 190°C (gas mark 5) for 15–20 minutes until lightly browned and cooked inside.

THAI GREEN CURRY IN A HURRY

This quick and easy family-friendly curry in a hurry is one of our favourite suppers. It's also super versatile. You can play with the spice level and swap out the chicken for prawns or tofu. To save time, make the curry paste in advance – it's so quick to whizz everything together. We've kept this dish slimming-friendly by using reduced-fat coconut milk, and we've upped the gut goodness with a selection of spices to aid digestion.

SERVES
2

PREP
15
minutes

COOK
15
minutes

470
kcals
PER SERVING

60g basmati rice (dry weight)
olive oil spray
200g chicken breast fillets, cut into strips
180ml canned reduced-fat coconut milk
3 kaffir lime leaves
80g mangetout, trimmed
a handful of basil, shredded
2 tbsp chopped pistachios
1–2 tsp lime or lemon juice
sea salt

For the Thai green curry paste
1 lemongrass stalk, peeled and sliced
½ small onion, sliced
2 green chillies
2cm piece of fresh root ginger, peeled
2 garlic cloves, peeled
small bunch of coriander
1 tsp coriander seeds, crushed
1 tsp black peppercorns
grated zest and juice of 1 lime
2 tsp nam pla (Thai fish sauce)

1. To make the Thai green curry paste, put all the ingredients into a blender or food processor and blitz to a paste.

2. Cook the rice according to the instructions on the packet.

3. Meanwhile, lightly spray a large frying pan with oil and set over a medium heat. Cook the chicken, turning occasionally, for 4–5 minutes until golden brown.

4. Add the Thai green curry paste and cook, stirring occasionally, for 2 minutes. Add the coconut milk and lime leaves, and simmer for 5 minutes more, then stir in the mangetout. Cook for another 3–4 minutes until the sauce thickens and the mangetout is just tender but still quite firm. Check the seasoning, adding salt to taste, and stir in the basil.

5. Stir the pistachios and lemon juice into the cooked rice, fluffing it up with a fork. Serve with the curry.

Tip
Double or quadruple the curry paste ingredients and store the leftover paste in a screw-top jar in the fridge for up to 2 weeks, or freeze it for up to 3 months.

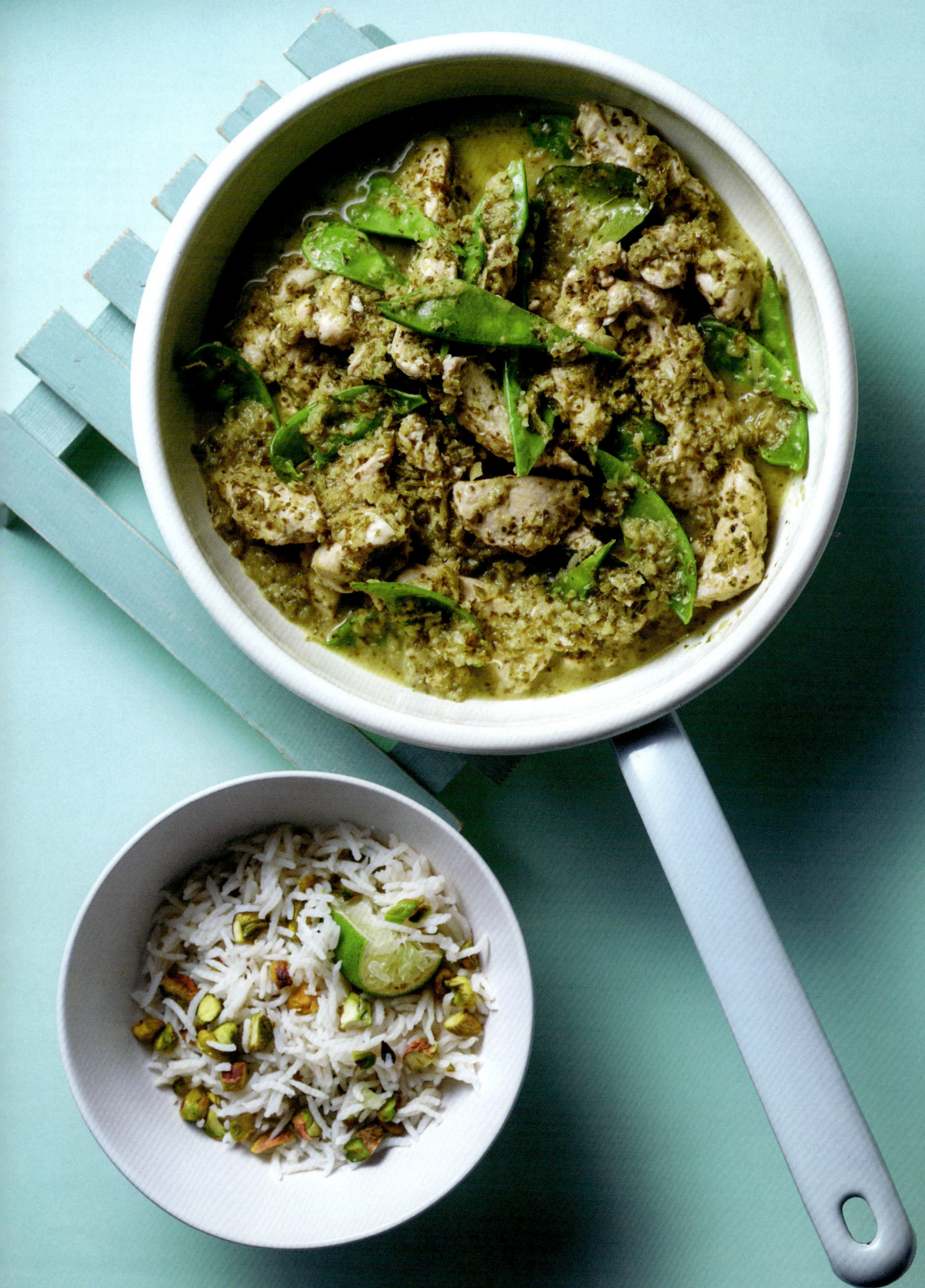

SPEEDY LAKSA with noodles

This is a spicy Southeast Asian dish of noodles, vegetables and chicken in a creamy coconut flavoured broth. It's a comforting, colourful bowl of goodness, with a satisfying energy boost from the noodles. You could double the quantities and keep the leftovers in the fridge for 2–3 days, reheating for an easy supper.

SERVES
2

PREP
15
minutes

COOK
15–20
minutes

400
kcals
PER SERVING

olive oil spray
4 spring onions, sliced
100g mushrooms, sliced
2 garlic cloves, crushed
2 tsp grated fresh root ginger
1 red chilli, finely sliced
1 lemongrass stalk, peeled and diced
1 tsp ground turmeric
400ml hot chicken stock
200ml reduced-fat coconut milk

1 tsp nam pla (Thai fish sauce)
200g cooked skinless chicken breast, sliced
60g rice noodles (dry weight)
80g long-stem broccoli, trimmed
50g bean sprouts
juice of 1 lime
a few coriander sprigs, chopped
sea salt and freshly ground black pepper

1. Lightly spray a pan with oil and set over a medium–high heat. Add the spring onions, mushrooms, garlic, ginger, chilli, lemongrass and turmeric, and stir-fry for 2–3 minutes. Add the hot stock, coconut milk and nam pla. Reduce the heat and simmer for 5 minutes, then add the chicken and simmer gently for another 5 minutes.

2. Meanwhile, cook the noodles according to the instructions on the packet and drain well.

3. Bring a pan of water to the boil, then reduce the heat to medium. Put the broccoli in a steamer basket over the pan, then cover and cook for 5 minutes, or until just tender.

4. Stir the rice noodles and bean sprouts into the laksa, and season to taste with salt and pepper. Heat through gently for 2–3 minutes, then stir in the lime juice.

5. Ladle the laksa into two shallow serving bowls, and top with the coriander and broccoli to serve.

Tip
To make this vegetarian, use vegetable stock or soy sauce instead of nam pla, and substitute tofu for the chicken.

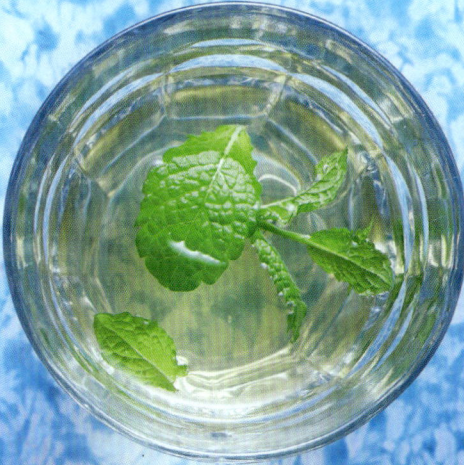

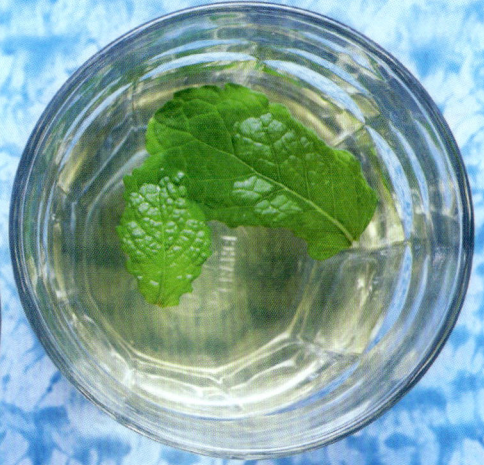

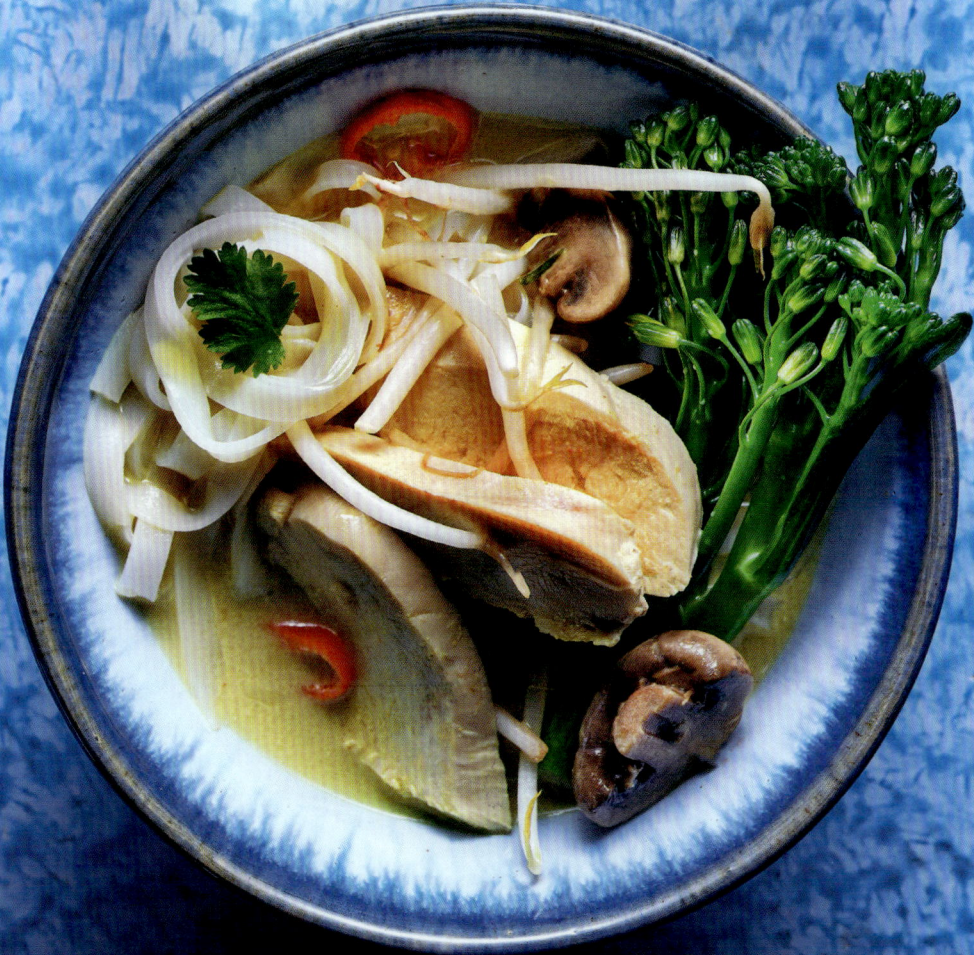

CHICKEN SOUVLAKI with tzatziki

Chicken souvlaki is a Greek classic: tender, marinated pieces of chicken served in a wrap with crispy salad leaves, juicy tomatoes and tzatziki. This is a delicious way to treat your body to a slimming, gut-healthy meal of protein, vitamins, minerals and fibre.

SERVES
2

PREP
10
minutes

CHILL
30
minutes

COOK
10
minutes

370
kcals
PER SERVING

250g skinned chicken breast fillets, cut into chunks
1 small red onion, peeled and cut into chunks
olive oil spray
2 wholemeal wraps (about 40g each)
a few crisp cos lettuce leaves, shredded
2 ripe tomatoes, sliced
handful of flat-leaf parsley, chopped

4 tbsp tzatziki (see Dairy-free Tzatziki, page 79)
smoked paprika, for dusting
sea salt and freshly ground black pepper

For the marinade
1 tsp fennel seeds
½ tsp dried oregano
1 garlic clove, crushed
grated zest and juice of 1 lemon
1 tsp olive oil

1. To make the marinade, crush the fennel seeds using a pestle and mortar, and transfer to a bowl. Add the oregano, garlic, lemon zest and juice, and oil, and stir to combine.

2. Thread the chicken and red onion on to 4 long bamboo skewers (see Tip). Place in a shallow dish and pour over the marinade. Cover and chill at least 30 minutes.

3. Preheat the grill to high. Lightly spray the skewers with oil and place on a foil-lined baking tray. Cook under the hot grill for 10 minutes, turning occasionally, until the chicken is golden brown and cooked right through, and the onion is tender. Alternatively, cook them in a ridged griddle pan over a medium–high heat, or over hot coals on a barbecue.

4. Warm the wraps in a hot griddle pan or a low oven. Divide the lettuce and tomatoes between each wrap, then remove the chicken and onions from the skewers and arrange on top. Sprinkle with parsley, then add tzatziki to each one and dust with paprika. Fold the wraps over the filling, and wrap in baking parchment to hold the filling in place. Enjoy!

Tip
To prevent the bamboo skewers scorching, soak them in water for 30 minutes before using.

SLOW-COOKED BEEF STEW
with root vegetables

On a chilly day, you can't beat a comforting hug-in-a-bowl stew, especially when the aromas are wafting through the door as you come home! We've used a slow cooker for this recipe, but you can just as easily pop it into the oven on a low heat (see note). Slow-cooking has a magical way of transforming the flavours and releasing the natural sweetness of the vegetables. We've chosen a selection here, because your gut loves diversity and each vegetable adds its own unique goodness. The wonderful thing about a slow cooker is you can prepare everything in advance and leave it to cook while you're busy doing other things.

SERVES
2

PREP
20
minutes

COOK
4
hours

400
kcals
PER SERVING

olive oil spray
1 small onion, finely sliced
2 celery sticks, chopped
1 large carrot, sliced
3 garlic cloves, crushed
225g lean stewing or braising steak, all visible fat removed, cubed
300g butternut squash, peeled, deseeded and cubed
150g swede, peeled and cubed
100g parsnips, peeled and cut into batons
350ml hot beef stock

200g canned chopped tomatoes
2 tsp tomato purée
1 tbsp Worcestershire sauce
1 bay leaf
2 thyme or rosemary sprigs
1 small juicy orange
100g dark green cabbage, shredded
handful of flat-leaf parsley, chopped
sea salt and freshly ground black pepper

1. Lightly spray a large pan with oil and set over a low heat. Add the onion, celery, carrot and garlic, and cook for 8–10 minutes, stirring occasionally, until tender. Remove and set aside.

2. Add the beef to the pan and cook over a medium heat, stirring often, for 5 minutes, or until browned all over. Stir in the squash, swede and parsnips, then add the hot stock, tomatoes and tomato purée, and bring to the boil. Reduce the heat and return the onion and carrot mixture to the pan, along with the Worcestershire sauce, bay leaf and thyme or rosemary.

continues overleaf

DINNERS

3. With a potato peeler, peel a long, wide strip of rind off the orange, then squeeze the juice. Add the juice and peel strip to the pan. Tip everything into the slow cooker, and cook on high for 4 hours or low for 7–8 hours. The vegetables should be tender and the beef falling apart.

4. Just before serving, cook the cabbage in a pan of boiling salted water for 4–5 minutes until bright green and just tender. Drain and season with salt and pepper.

5. Remove the herb sprigs from the stew and season to taste with salt and pepper. Serve immediately with the cabbage, with parsley sprinkled on top.

Tip
This is also great served with broccoli or carrots.

NOTES
This freezes well, so you could make double the quantity and freeze half. Defrost thoroughly before reheating.
Conventional cooking: Use a flameproof casserole dish instead of a large saucepan and slow cooker. Cook in a preheated oven at 160°C (gas mark 3 for 2–3 hours) until the meat is tender and the liquid has reduced.

STEAK & CHIPS with chimichurri

If there was only one sauce we could bring on our desert island get-away, it would be chimichurri! This tangy, garlicky, herby addition transforms any meal from ordinary to extraordinary. Flavour-wise it's fantastic, but we also love it for the many health-boosting benefits hidden in the herbs, garlic, vinegar, olive oil and chilli.

SERVES
2

PREP
15
minutes

COOK
20
minutes

370
kcals
PER SERVING

200g sweet potato, peeled and cut into thin chips
olive oil spray
2 fillet or sirloin steaks (about 100g each), all visible fat removed
sea salt and freshly ground black pepper

juice of ½ lemon
1 small red chilli, diced
¼ tsp smoked paprika
1 garlic clove, crushed
handful of coriander, chopped
handful of flat-leaf parsley, chopped
a few mint sprigs, chopped

For the chimichurri sauce
1 tbsp olive oil
1 tsp red wine vinegar

To serve
8 baby plum tomatoes
green salad

1. To make the chimichurri sauce, combine all the ingredients in a bowl. Blitz with a stick blender, and season to taste with salt and pepper.

2. Preheat the oven to 190°C (gas mark 5).

3. Lightly spray the sweet potato chips with oil and season with salt and pepper. Spread them out on a baking tray and cook in the preheated oven for 20 minutes, or until crisp and golden brown.

4. Meanwhile, spray the steaks lightly with oil and season with salt and pepper. Set a ridged griddle pan over a medium–high heat and, when it's hot, add the steaks. Cook for 2–4 minutes on each side, depending on how you like your steak. Ideally, they should be slightly charred on the outside and juicy and pink inside. Set aside to rest for 4–5 minutes.

5. Place a steak on each plate and spoon over the chimichurri sauce. Serve with the hot sweet potato fries and some tomatoes and green salad.

Tip
You can make healthy vegetable chips in the same way with swede or butternut squash.

DINNERS

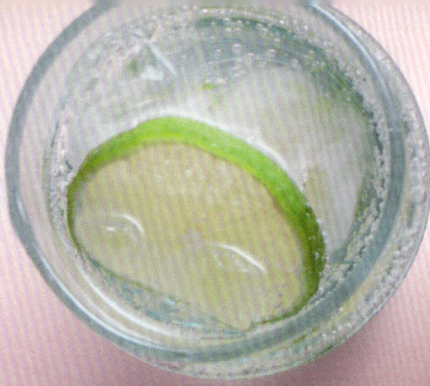

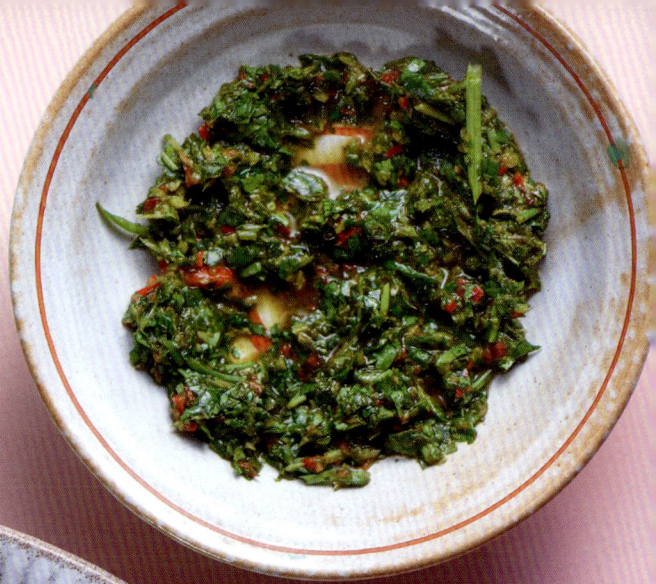

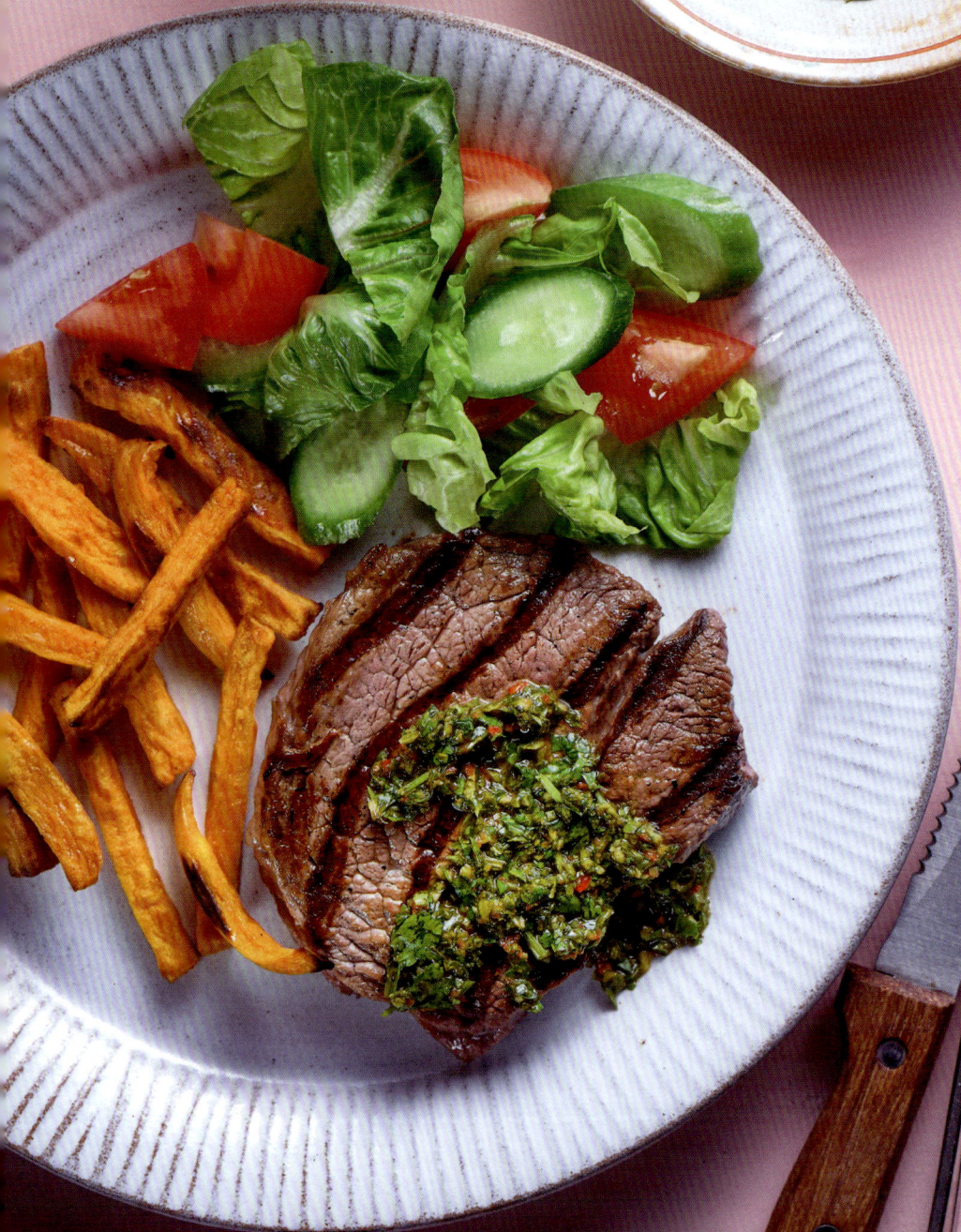

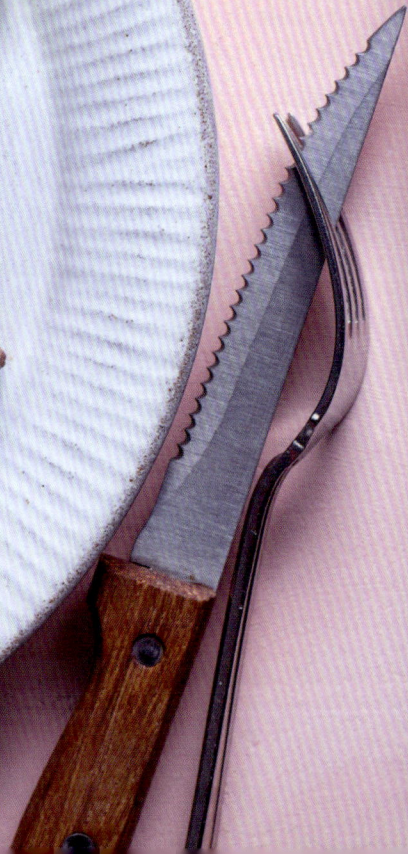

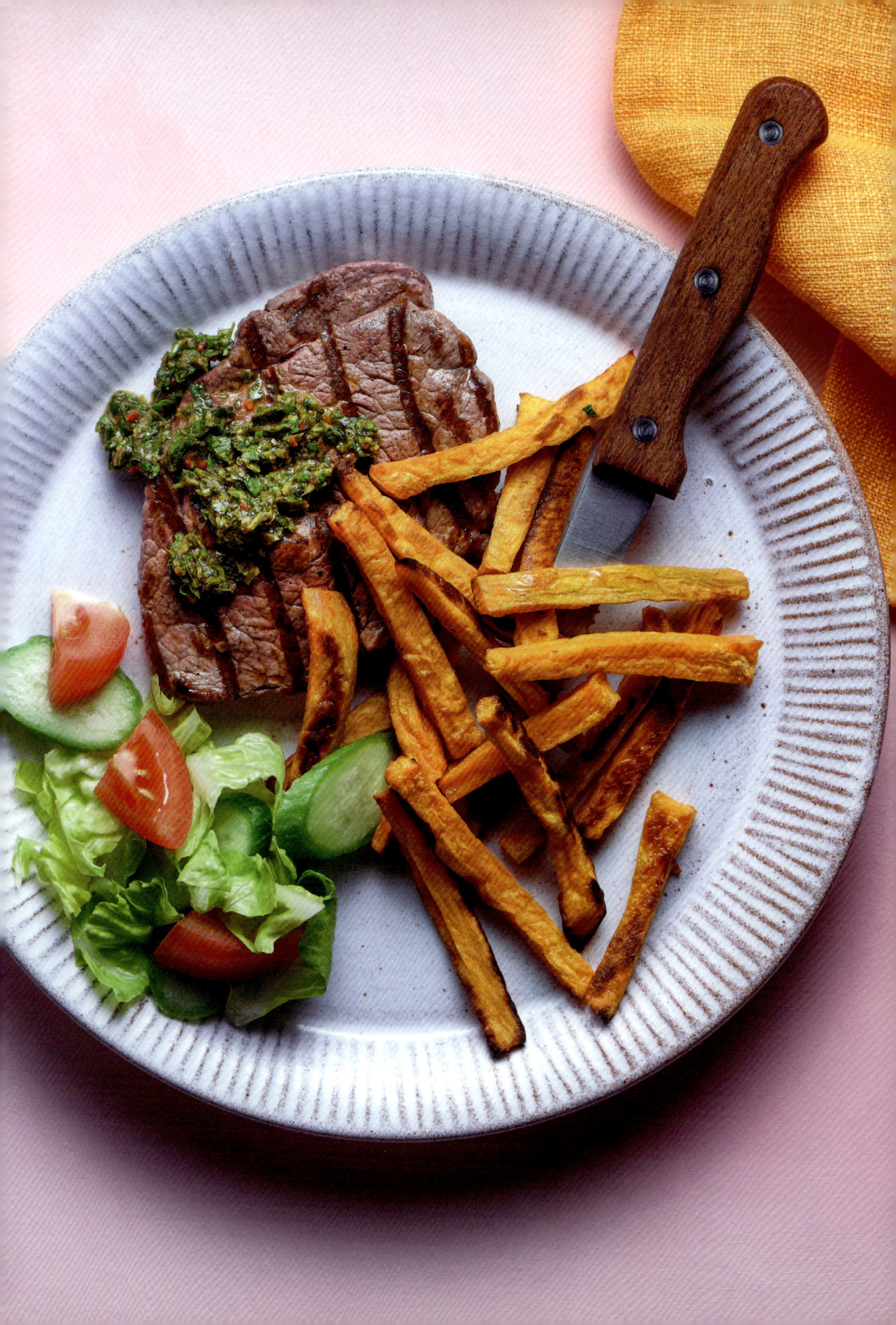

CREAMY BEEF STROGANOFF

We've given the classic beef stroganoff a super-healthy, slimming twist by using reduced-fat cream, very lean steak and wholemeal pasta, while mushrooms bring their gut-loving goodness to the party. The delicious creamy sauce is full of good-gut friends, such as mustard, Greek yogurt and a sprinkling of paprika. This is another quick supper dish, ready in less than 30 minutes, and extremely nourishing.

SERVES
2

PREP
10
minutes

COOK
15
minutes

430
kcals
PER SERVING

2 tsp olive oil
1 small onion, finely sliced
200g mushrooms, thickly sliced
1 tsp Dijon mustard
dash of Worcestershire sauce
250g lean rump or fillet steak, all visible fat removed, sliced into thin strips
2 tbsp reduced-fat crème fraîche
60g fat-free Greek yogurt
handful of flat-leaf parsley, finely chopped
60g tagliatelle or fettuccine (dry weight), preferably wholewheat
80g broccoli florets
paprika, for dusting
sea salt and freshly ground black pepper

1. Heat the oil in a frying pan set over a medium heat. Add the onion and cook for 5 minutes, or until softened, then add the mushrooms and cook, stirring occasionally, for 2–3 minutes until starting to brown. Stir in the mustard and Worcestershire sauce to taste.

2. Add the steak and cook for 3–5 minutes more, depending on how well done you like it. Lower the heat to a bare simmer and stir in the crème fraîche and yogurt. Heat through very gently, then season to taste and stir in the parsley.

3. Meanwhile, cook the pasta according to the instructions on the packet. Drain well.

4. At the same time, bring a pan of water to the boil, then reduce the heat to medium. Put the broccoli in a steamer basket over the pan, then cover and cook for 5 minutes, or until just tender.

5. Serve the pasta and steamed broccoli with the creamy beef and mushrooms, dusted with paprika.

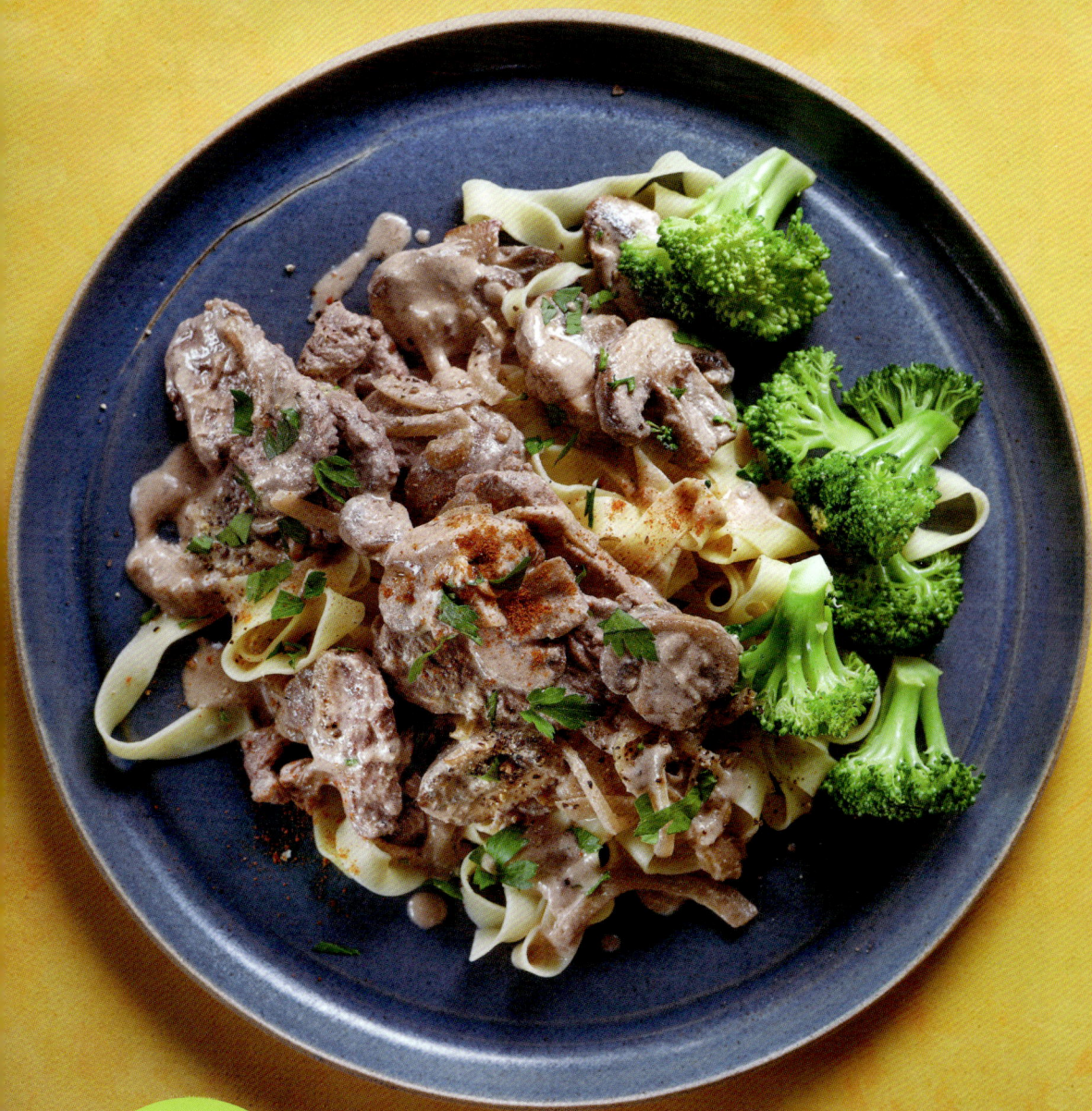

Tip
If you don't have broccoli, this is delicious with any green vegetables or a salad.

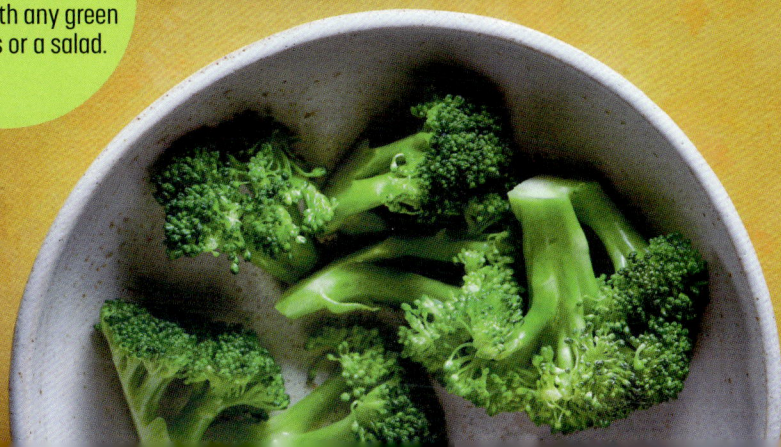

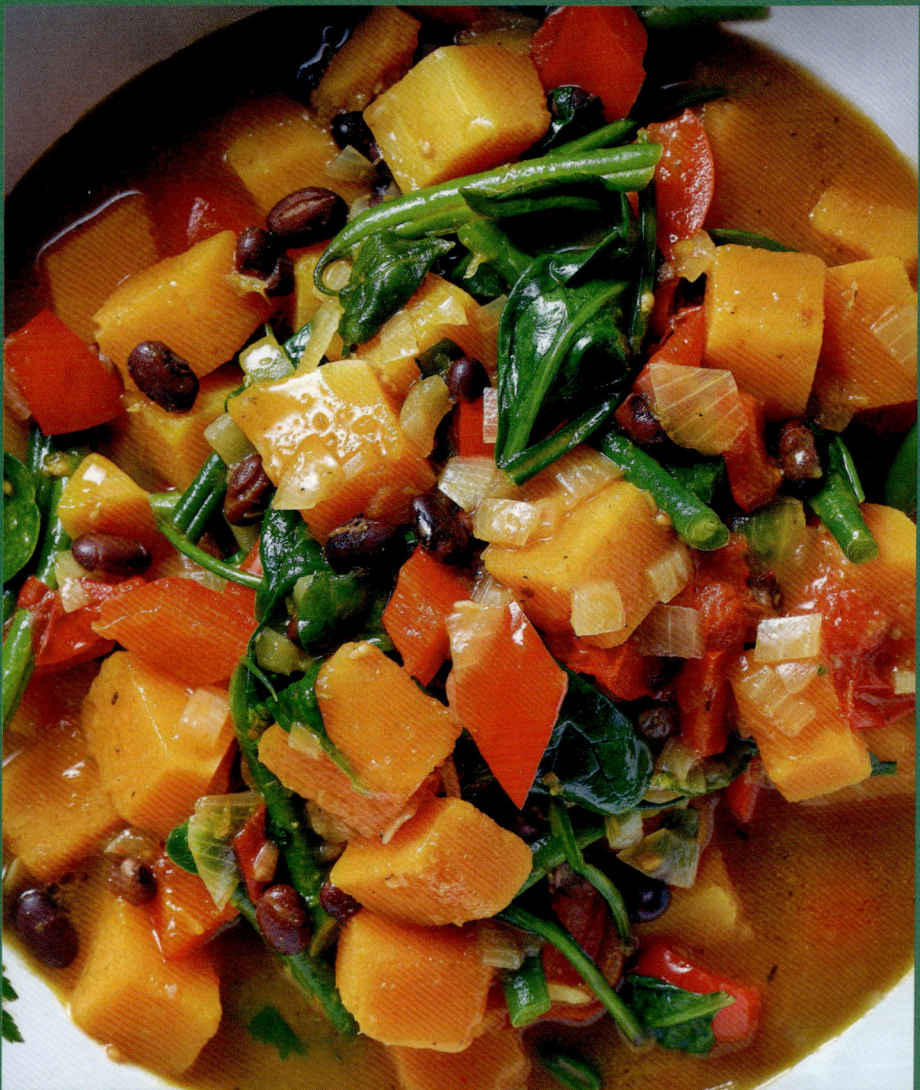

CRISPY TOFU STIR-FRY

This super-fast stir-fry features crispy tofu as the star ingredient. Tofu is a fantastic plant-based protein. It's also very easy to cook, but because it has a mild taste, it needs to be marinated first or cooked with strong flavours. We've given this stir-fry a spicy kick, added lots of fresh vegetables for a pop of colour, and tossed in some noodles for a sustained energy boost.

SERVES
2

PREP
10
minutes

COOK
10–12
minutes

430
kcals
PER SERVING

200g firm or extra-firm tofu, drained, pressed and cubed (see note)
2 tsp cornflour
1 tsp sesame oil
4 spring onions, finely sliced
2 garlic cloves, crushed
1 red chilli, finely sliced
2cm piece of fresh root ginger, peeled and diced
1 red or yellow pepper, sliced

80g mangetout or sugar snap peas, trimmed
200g spring greens, kale or spinach, sliced
150g straight-to-wok rice noodles
1 tbsp soy sauce
juice of 1 lime
2 tbsp roasted cashew nuts
sea salt and freshly ground black pepper

1. Dust the tofu with the cornflour and season with salt and pepper. Heat the sesame oil in a wok or frying pan set over a medium–high heat, and stir-fry the tofu for 4–5 minutes until crisp and golden brown. Remove and drain on a plate lined with kitchen paper. Keep warm.

2, Reduce the heat to medium and add the spring onions, garlic, chilli and ginger to the pan. Stir-fry for 1 minute, then add the pepper and mangetout or sugar snap peas, and stir-fry for 2–3 minutes more. Stir in the greens and noodles and continue to cook for 2–3 minutes until the vegetables are just tender but still retain some bite. Toss in the soy sauce and lime juice.

3. Serve immediately, topped with the crispy tofu and cashews.

NOTES
To press tofu, remove it from the pack and drain off any liquid. Cut into thick slices and place them between 2 sheets of kitchen paper on a plate. Cover with a clean cloth and put a heavy weight, such as cans or books, on top. After 30 minutes, drain, pat dry with kitchen paper and cut into cubes.

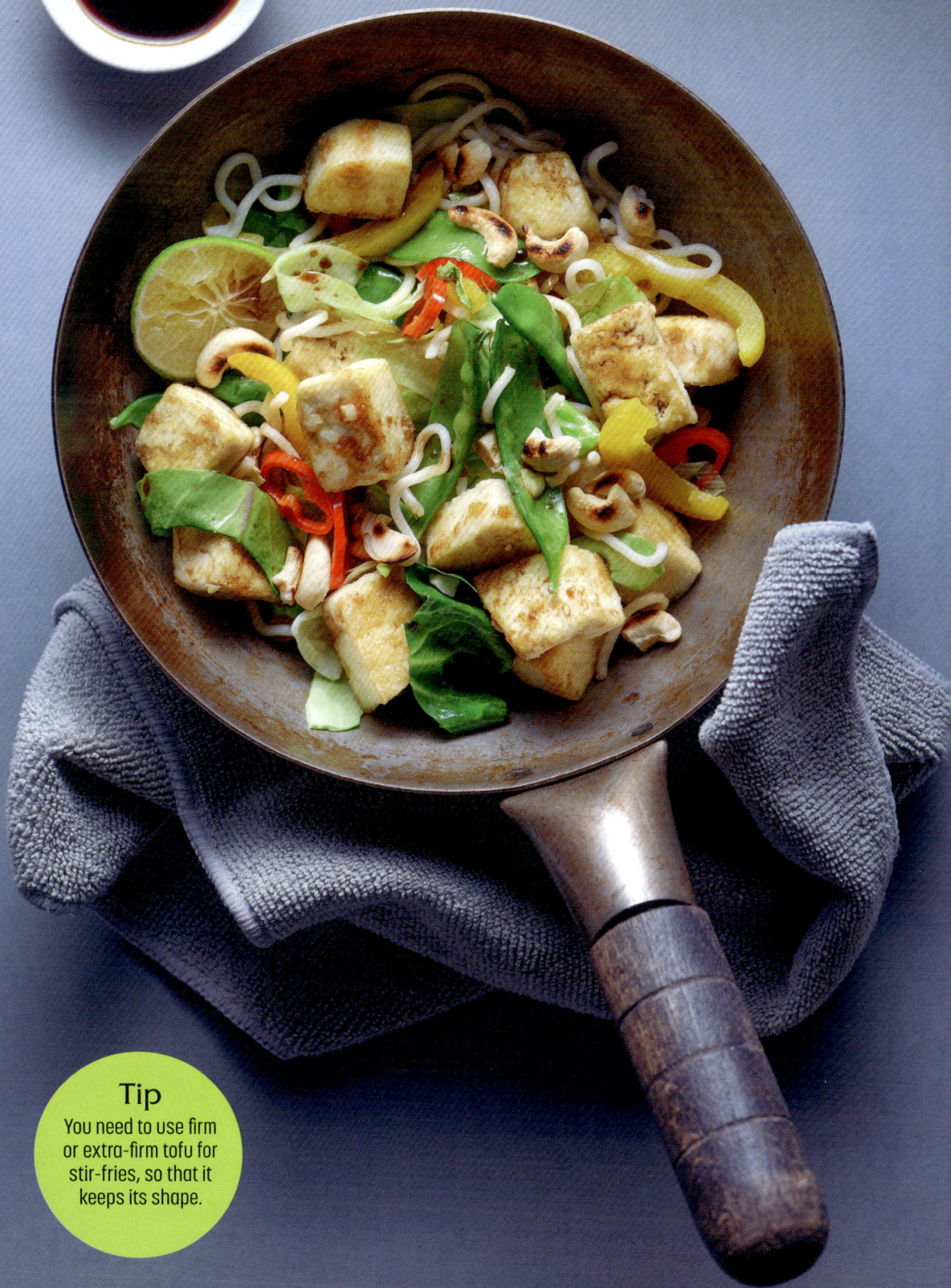

Tip
You need to use firm or extra-firm tofu for stir-fries, so that it keeps its shape.

5. Stir the rice into the onion mixture and cook until all the grains are glistening and so hot that they start to crackle. Quickly pour in the wine and cook until the liquid evaporates. Reduce the heat to a simmer and add a ladleful of the stock. Stir gently until all the liquid is absorbed, then add another ladleful. Keep doing this, one ladleful at a time, until most or all of the stock has been absorbed and the rice grains are plump and tender, but still retain a little 'bite' – they should not be soft and mushy. This will take about 15 minutes.

6. Remove from the heat and gently stir in the spinach purée and torn basil, along with most of the grated Parmesan and lemon juice. Season to taste and serve immediately, sprinkled with the remaining Parmesan.

Tip
You don't have to add wine, but it will enhance the flavour of the risotto.

NOTE
For best results, use fresh spinach and good-quality vegetable stock.

VEGAN KATSU CURRY

Here's a delicious homemade version of the popular Japanese curry. We've used an air fryer to reduce the oil used and make the panko aubergine fritters healthier, but there are instructions in the tip below for conventional cooking. Instead of beaten egg, we've used drained canned chickpea liquid (aquafaba) for the crispy coating.

SERVES
2

PREP
15
minutes

DRAIN
30
minutes

COOK
15–18
minutes

350
kcals
PER SERVING

olive oil spray
1 small red onion, chopped
3 garlic cloves, crushed
1 carrot, diced
2cm piece of fresh root ginger, grated
1–2 tsp mild curry powder
1 tsp ground turmeric
1 tbsp tomato purée
120ml canned reduced-fat coconut milk
60g brown rice (dry weight)

lime wedges, for squeezing

For the panko aubergine fritters

1 large aubergine, sliced into 5mm rounds
large pinch of salt
2 tbsp plain flour
3 tbsp aquafaba (the liquid from a can of chickpeas)
40g panko breadcrumbs

1. Begin by making the panko aubergine fritters. Place the aubergine rounds in a colander standing in the sink. Sprinkle with the salt and set aside for 30 minutes to drain; the salt will draw out excess moisture. Pat the slices dry with kitchen paper and dust with the flour.

2. Preheat the air fryer to 190°C.

3. Dip the aubergine slices into the aquafaba, and then coat all over with the panko breadcrumbs. Spray lightly with oil on both sides, then arrange them in a single layer in the air fryer basket (you may have to do this in batches, depending on the size of your air fryer). Cook for 15–18 minutes, turning halfway, until golden brown and crispy.

continues overleaf

CREAMY GARLIC MUSHROOM GNOCCHI

We've given this creamy gnocchi dish a healthy makeover by swapping high-fat ingredients for some slimmer alternatives. It's quick and easy to make, and it's full of nourishing goodness. Mushrooms are your gut's best buddy! These fungi friends promote the growth of good bacteria, supporting your overall health and immunity.

SERVES
2

PREP
10
minutes

COOK
15
minutes

390
kcals
PER SERVING

olive oil spray
1 onion, finely chopped
1 leek, finely sliced
3 garlic cloves, crushed
250g chestnut mushrooms, sliced or quartered
100ml vegetable stock
4 tbsp reduced-fat crème fraîche

100g baby spinach leaves
2 tbsp toasted pine nuts
200g potato gnocchi
a few flat-leaf parsley sprigs, chopped
2 tbsp grated Parmesan cheese
sea salt and freshly ground black pepper

1. Lightly spray a large frying pan with oil and set over a medium heat. Add the onion, leek and garlic, and cook for 5 minutes, stirring occasionally, until tender. Add the mushrooms and cook for 5 minutes more until golden brown. Season lightly with salt and pepper.

2. Add the stock and increase the heat to high. When it starts to boil, reduce the heat and simmer for 5 minutes, or until the sauce reduces. Stir in the crème fraîche, spinach and pine nuts, and cook for 2 minutes more, or until the spinach wilts into the sauce. Season with salt and pepper.

3. Meanwhile, cook the gnocchi in a pan of boiling water according to the packet instructions. Drain well.

4. Stir the cooked gnocchi into the mushroom sauce and serve immediately in shallow bowls, sprinkled with parsley and grated Parmesan.

Tip
You can use any mushrooms you prefer, even wild ones if it's a special occasion.

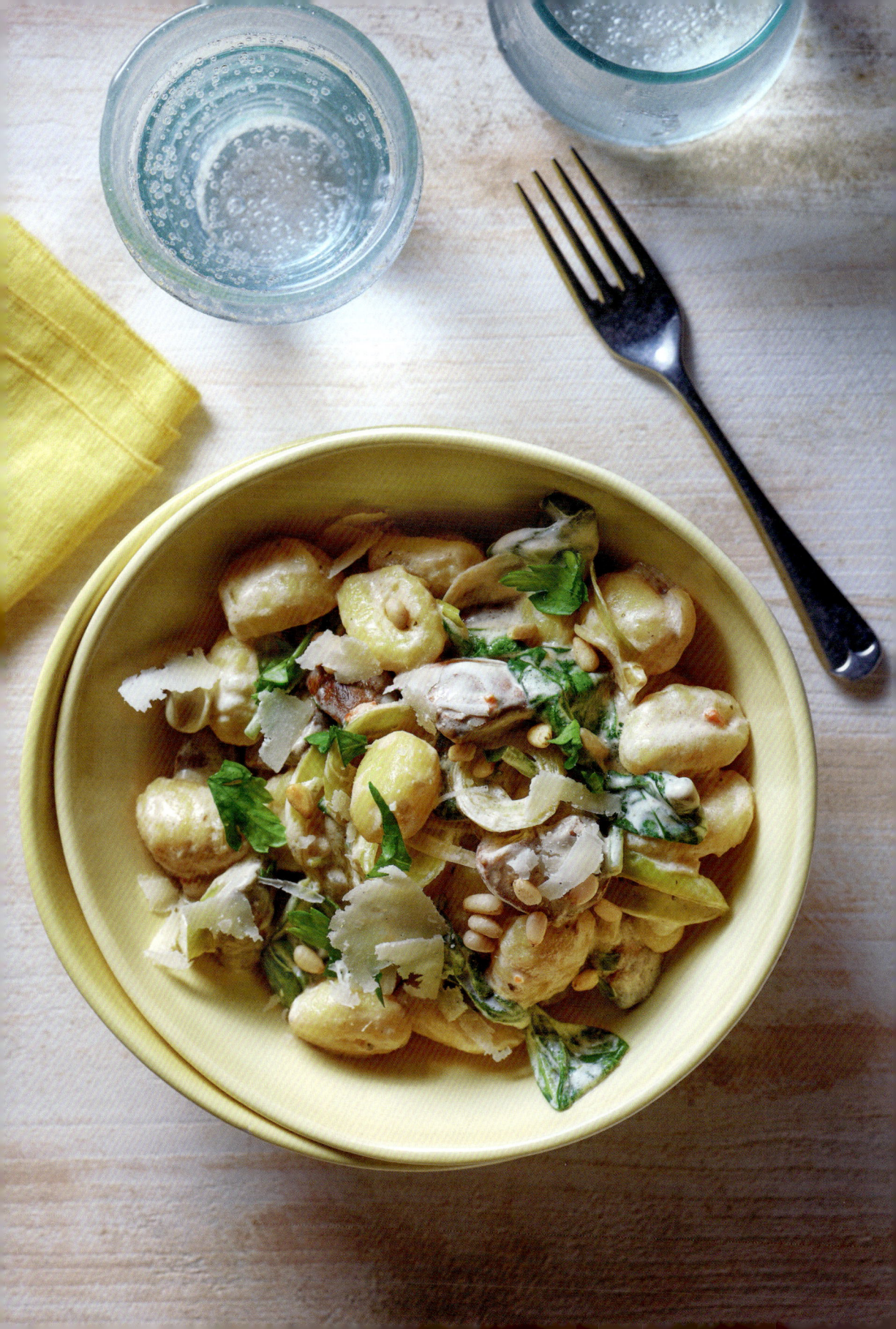

CARIBBEAN-STYLE RAINBOW CURRY

This colourful one-pot vegetable curry is full of flavour and goodness. You can buy West Indian or Caribbean curry paste in many supermarkets and delis, as well as online. Alternately, just use ½ teaspoon each of the following anti-inflammatory ground spices: turmeric, ginger, cinnamon, cumin, coriander, nutmeg, allspice and cayenne pepper.

SERVES
2

PREP
15
minutes

COOK
30
minutes

420
kcals
PER SERVING

olive oil spray
1 onion, diced
1 red pepper, cubed
2 garlic cloves, crushed
1 red chilli, diced
1 tsp ground turmeric
1–2 tsp West Indian or Caribbean curry paste
200ml canned reduced-fat coconut milk
75ml hot vegetable stock
1 cinnamon stick

300g pumpkin, peeled, deseeded and cubed
200g canned black beans, drained and rinsed
80g fine green beans, trimmed and halved
8 cherry or baby plum tomatoes, halved
juice of 1 lime
80g baby spinach leaves
handful of coriander, chopped
60g basmati rice (dry weight)
sea salt and freshly ground black pepper

1. Lightly spray a pan with oil and set over a low–medium heat. Add the onion and red pepper and cook, stirring occasionally, for 6–8 minutes until softened. Stir in the garlic and chilli and cook for 2 minutes more, then add the turmeric and curry paste. Cook for another 1–2 minutes.

2. Add the coconut milk, stock, cinnamon stick and pumpkin. Cover the pan and cook for 10 minutes before adding the black beans, green beans and tomatoes. Simmer for 10 minutes until all the vegetables are tender.

3. Stir in the lime juice, spinach and most of the coriander. Cook gently for another 2–3 minutes, or until the spinach wilts into the curry. Season to taste and remove the cinnamon stick.

4. Cook the rice according to the instructions on the packet. Spoon the curry into two bowls, sprinkle with the remaining coriander, and serve with the rice.

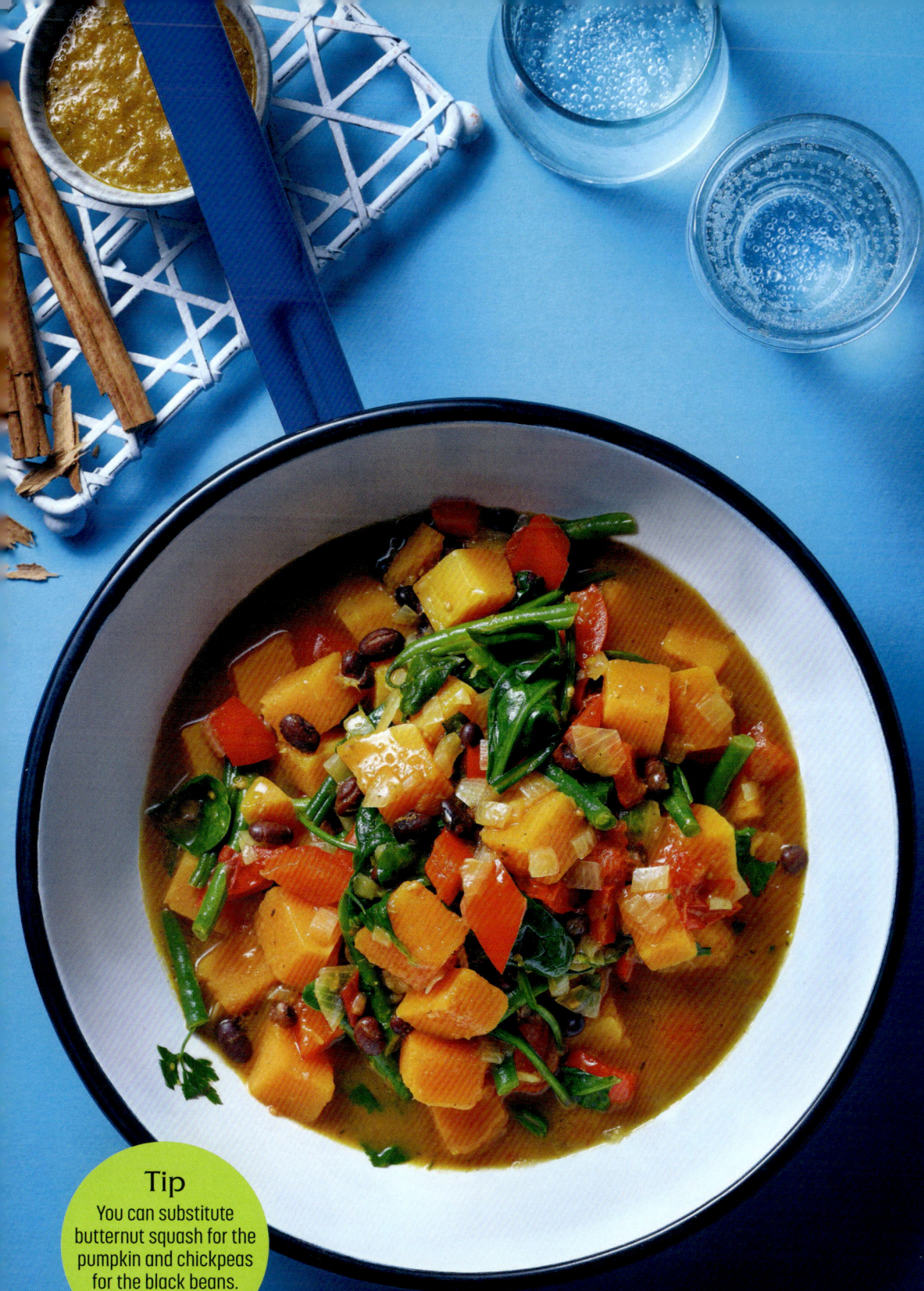

Tip
You can substitute butternut squash for the pumpkin and chickpeas for the black beans.

OUR STORY

It was a sales assistant, a local priest and a school teacher who inspired Agnes McCourt to change her life and find her passion in the world of health and fitness.

This is the story of Unislim.

It all began with a chance encounter in the late 1960s. While shopping for a dress for a glamorous party, a sales assistant crushed Agnes's enthusiasm, telling her nothing would fit, but she 'might find a dress in the maternity section'. Agnes left the shop in tears. Deflated but not defeated, she went home determined to do something.

Tears quickly turned to cups of tea and talk over the kitchen table. Her husband Brian, a teacher, suggested she rally a group of friends to support each other, learn how to eat more healthily and motivate each other to get fit. Agnes's local priest insisted she use the community hall for the group and, before she knew it, she had the keys, an idea and eight willing friends.

Back then, there were no mobile phones, computers, gyms or fitness clubs. With very few sources of information, Brian dusted down the Encyclopaedia Britannica and studied up on nutrition to find weekly topics for the group to discuss. Agnes used her knowledge as a PE teacher to inspire and motivate her friends to exercise and adopt healthier habits. It worked. Soon the small group of women all reached their desired weight. But, more importantly, they felt amazing. The local paper caught wind of 'the woman who could talk the weight off you' and Agnes became a news sensation.

Agnes and Brian saw an opportunity, not just to change their lives, but to ignite a broader movement. With three young children, they took a leap of faith, gave up their jobs and followed their passion.

What started around a kitchen table soon grew into a nationwide phenomenon. Unislim became a household name with a strong community spirit that brought people together to achieve common wellness goals. The company's ethos – rooted in empathy, education, and encouragement – continues to inspire thousands of people to make positive lifestyle changes through a network of weekly meetings and online courses.

Evolving with scientifically backed nutritional knowledge, Unislim remains holistic in its approach. We understand how stress, lack of sleep and lifestyle factors can affect eating habits and encourage our community to view all aspects of their life in order to make healthy changes. At Unislim, food is a friend to be celebrated and enjoyed.

Brian passed away at the age of 48, while Agnes continued running classes and inspiring members until the 2000s. Her daughter Fiona is now CEO and her grandchildren Luca, a fitness instructor, and Mila, a yoga teacher, are also following in her footsteps.

We created this book with love and hope you find it engaging, inspiring and educational. Best wishes to you to live a fulfilled, happy and healthy life.

Unislim x

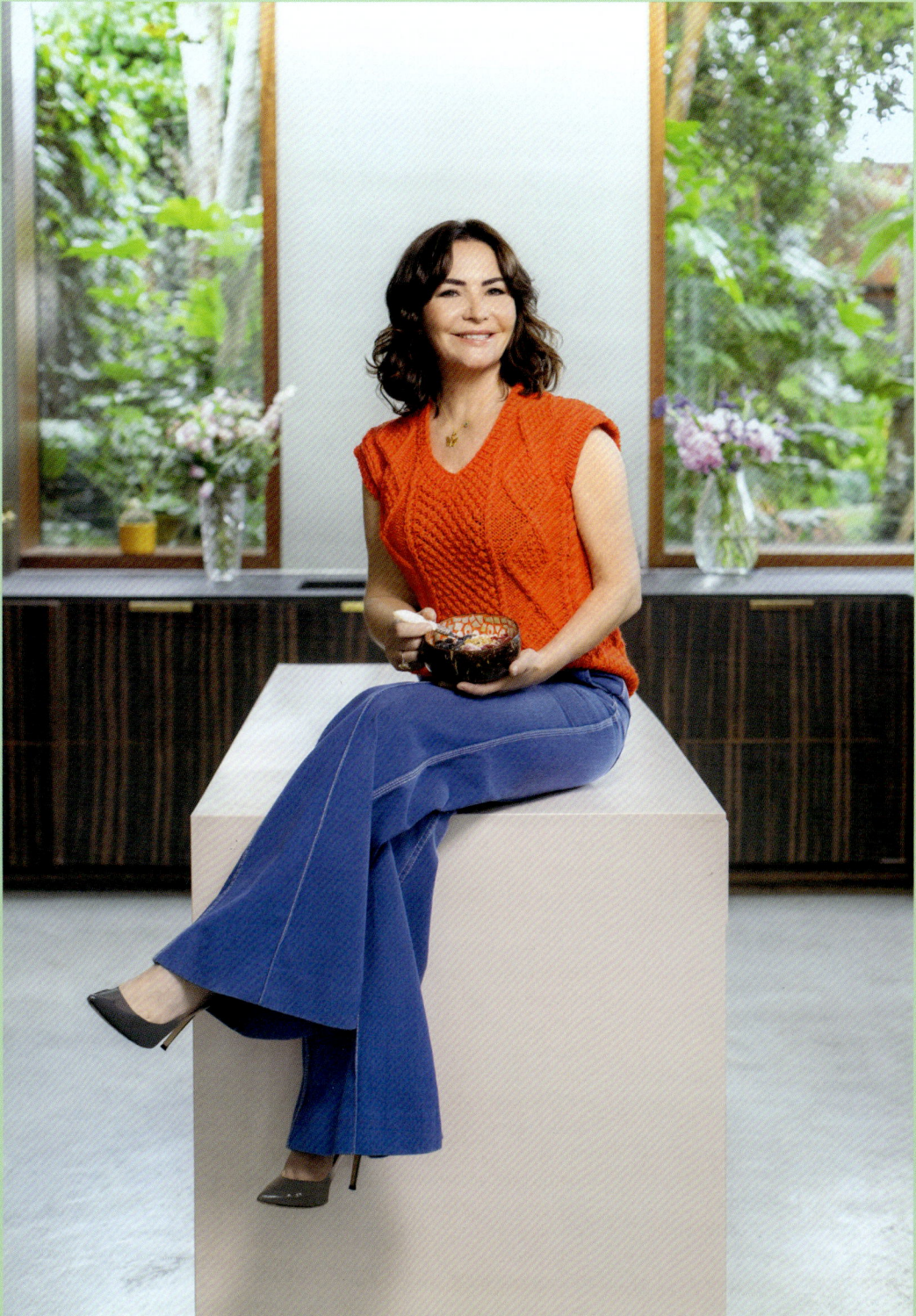

INDEX

1

Published in 2024 by Ebury Press, an imprint of Ebury Publishing
Penguin Random House UK
One Embassy Gardens, 8 Viaduct Gdns,
Nine Elms, London SW11 7BW

Ebury Press is part of the Penguin Random House group of companies whose addresses
can be found at global.penguinrandomhouse.com

Penguin
Random House
UK

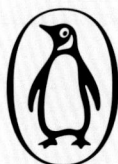

Text © Ebury Press
Photography © Ebury Press
Design © Ebury Press

Fiona Gratzer has asserted her right to be identified as the author of this Work in accordance
with the Copyright, Designs and Patents Act 1988

Penguin Random House values and supports copyright. Copyright fuels creativity,
encourages diverse voices, promotes freedom of expression and supports a vibrant culture.
Thank you for purchasing an authorized edition of this book and for respecting intellectual
property laws by not reproducing, scanning or distributing any part of it by any means
without permission. You are supporting authors and enabling Penguin Random House to
continue to publish books for everyone. No part of this book may be used or reproduced
in any manner for the purpose of training artificial intelligence technologies or systems.
In accordance with Article 4(3) of the DSM Directive 2019/790, Penguin Random House
expressly reserves this work from the text and data mining exception.

First published by Ebury Press in 2024

www.penguin.co.uk

A CIP catalogue record for this book is available from the British Library

ISBN 9781529944327

Recipe Writer: Heather Thomas
Design: maru studio G.K.
Photography: Joff Lee Studios
Production: Percie Bridgewater
Publishing Director: Elizabeth Bond
Copy Editor: Tara O'Sullivan
Food stylist Mari Williams

The authorized representative in the EEA is Penguin Random House Ireland, Morrison
Chambers, 32 Nassau Street, Dublin, D02 YH68

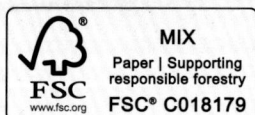

MIX
Paper | Supporting
responsible forestry
FSC® C018179
FSC
www.fsc.org

Penguin Random House is committed to a sustainable future for
our business, our readers and our planet. This book is made from
Forest Stewardship Council® certified paper.

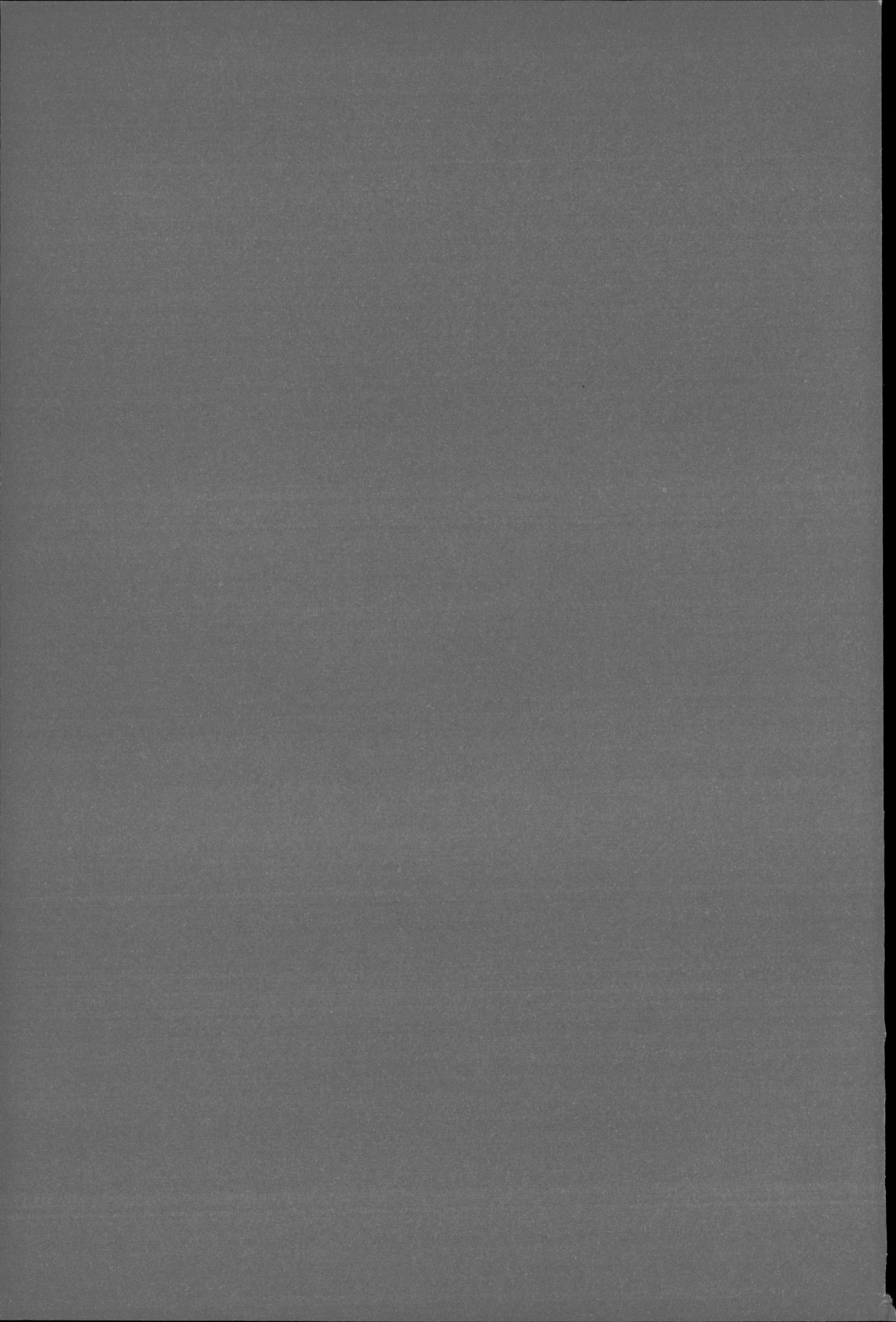